White Gold

....

Anthropology of Contemporary North America

SERIES EDITORS

James Bielo, *Miami University*

Carrie Lane, *California State University, Fullerton*

ADVISORY BOARD

Peter Benson, *Washington University in St. Louis*

John L. Caughey, *University of Maryland*

Alyshia Gálvez, *Lehman College*

Carol Greenhouse, *Princeton University*

John Hartigan, *University of Texas*

John Jackson Jr., *University of Pennsylvania*

Ellen Lewin, *University of Iowa*

Bonnie McElhinny, *University of Toronto*

Shalini Shankar, *Northwestern University*

Carol Stack, *University of California, Berkeley*

White Gold

Stories of Breast Milk Sharing

Susan Falls

University of Nebraska Press
Lincoln and London

Library of Congress Cataloging-in-Publication Data
Names: Falls, Susan.
Title: White gold: stories of breast milk sharing /
Susan Falls.
Description: Lincoln: University of Nebraska Press [2017] |
Series: Anthropology of contemporary North America |
Includes bibliographical references and index.
Identifiers: LCCN 2016054690 (print)
LCCN 2017000735 (ebook)
ISBN 9780803277212 (cloth: alk. paper)
ISBN 9781496201898 (pbk.: alk. paper)
ISBN 9781496202697 (epub)
ISBN 9781496202703 (mobi)
ISBN 9781496202710 (pdf)
Subjects: LCSH: Breastfeeding. |
Breastfeeding—Complications. | Breast milk.
Classification: LCC RJ216 .F3527 2017 (print) |
LCC RJ216 (ebook) | DDC 649/.33—dc23
LC record available at https://lccn.loc.gov/2016054690

Set in Charter ITC by Rachel Gould.

For my mother and all mothers

Contents

Illustrations

Preface

My son has more than twenty-five siblings—milk siblings, that is. I first learned of milk siblings not by reading about kinship with my Anthropology 101 class but by attending a presentation at the 2010 Visual Research Conference. A group of young women scholars and their professor, Fadwa El Guindi, discussed various ways that people reckon kinship in Qatar. Milk siblingship—when a child receives breast milk from a woman who is not the child's biological mother and thus enters into a kin relationship with her and her family—is practiced in many parts of the world. I was surprised and very excited to hear this.

Just a few weeks earlier, after having adopted a baby, I learned from my doula that if I was unable to breastfeed our son, I might be able to use donated breast milk. Many people around me were breastfeeding their children, and there seemed to be a general consensus that breast milk was better than formula. So I called the closest milk bank to inquire about getting some milk. To my great dismay I discovered that human milk is extremely expensive—all told, it would be almost six dollars per ounce. Since newborns consume about two to three ounces every four hours and older babies take up to six or eight ounces every six hours, the cost would be exorbitant. Unless, I thought, my insurance would pay for it. I phoned my medical provider and made an inquiry.

"Do you know if there is a generic brand of this medication?" the woman in customer service kept asking me. "No, it's not a pharmaceutical product," I replied. "It's breast milk, you know, from a breast—it does not have a generic brand name. I want to order it from the WakeMed Milk Bank with a prescription from our pediatrician." This situation was evidently one that her scripted answers to frequently asked questions did not cover. No matter how hard I tried I could not get her to understand my question: did our insurance policy cover the purchase of banked breast milk? It turned out to be a dead end. And there was no way we could spend that kind of money out of pocket every day. That experience did tell me, however, that what I was doing was out of the ordinary.

Serendipitously my doula—a birth facilitator—called that very afternoon to tell me about breast milk sharing. She had met the coordinator of a local milk-sharing group and wanted to introduce us. The group, all volunteer, uses an online forum to help donors find people who need breast milk. Women who have milk to give post information about themselves, the age of their child, the kind of freezer they have, where they are located, and so forth. It is not uncommon for new mothers to store breast milk for later use but then find that they do not need it. Sometimes their child will not "take a bottle" and they decide to donate the milk rather than throw it out. It is after all a precious, life-giving substance that has taken time and energy for them to produce and store. Lactating mothers may provide a one-time donation, large or small, or they may always have extra milk to share and thus become regular, long-term donors.

Parents seeking milk also provide information, sometimes including detailed narratives about why they need it. Sometimes these accounts include explanations about cancer or other medical conditions that hinder milk production, or they discuss the trials and tribulations faced in having or trying to have children (adoptions, failed fertility treatments, miscarriages, severely premature babies, twins or triplets, or prenatal drug exposure). They often refer to breast milk itself with value-giving names, such as "white gold" or "liquid gold."

Once a match is made, donors and donees (who are of course acting as proxies for their babies) negotiate additional medical or personal questions they feel need to be addressed. My local group's coordinator, Ashley, provided me with a questionnaire that I was to give to potential donors. These questions helped me to understand the diet, lifestyle, and possible drug or disease exposures donors may have experienced.

I was amazed by how effectively this self-organized network functions. Except for when our son was just born (he drank formula until I got my network up and running, which took me about two weeks), he was fed breast milk until the age of eighteen months. Our adopted daughter also received donated breast milk until she was a bit more than a year old. Neither child, aged three and five in 2016, has experienced much in the way of sickness, which donors and doulas explain as a benefit of receiving antibodies from so many different families.

When I was new to the group I heard that although new mothers probably could make a handsome extra income, it is illegal to buy and sell breast milk. But when I looked into it I discovered that, for the time being, peer-to-peer milk shares are not overseen or regulated by the federal or state governments or by any other agency. A donee might offer the donor something in return for milk, and indeed in our case we often gave donors pumping supplies or flowers but never money. These offerings seemed to be appreciated but were neither required nor necessarily expected.

But back to milk siblings.

When we picked up the milk from one of our first donors, she asked for a photo and the full name of our son and provided us with the same, explaining, "Now that the children are milk siblings, we will need to know these things." In my ignorance I thought Anuka, an architect from Egypt who was living in Atlanta with her husband and two children, was just trying to be kind by finding a way to sentimentalize or just normalize what seemed like a pretty odd situation. How charming, I thought, and I sent her a specially selected photo of our baby. Little did I know that she was drawing on a venerable cultural tradition of "nurture kinship" whereby even strangers can be transformed into kin (and vice versa), a concept very different than that of kinship by blood, an ideology that despite anthropological critiques by Schneider (1968) and others remains hegemonic in the United States.

According to the Qatari women's presentation at the Visual Research Conference, the Quran explains the role and obligations of milk siblings in no less than three places (El Guindi 2011). Islamic law allows for women to cross-breastfeed babies, who may then become their children's relatives, with all that entails (for example, veiling customs, rules about who one can marry, and even inheritance or property rights). Other research shows milk siblingship to be "a strikingly widespread phenomenon, practiced by peoples from the Balkans to Bengal, from Marrakech to Mandalay," that creates lasting connections, shapes social distance from one group to another, and can be used to control others' behavior (MacClancy 2003). On my way to the airport after the conference my cabbie, an Egyptian named Fadil, confirmed that although the practice seems to be less common in some places, milk siblingship is still alive and well in Egypt, at least among his people. When I returned home I found a post on Juan Cole's blog *Informed Comment* that went beyond what Fadil had explained: Cole (2010) argues that Saudi clerics who are promoting kinship by sharing breast milk, while tinkering with the rules of traditional milk siblingship to apply to adults instead of children under the age of five, are doing so as a sign of modernization—not conservatism—in order to allow non-kin women and men to congregate. So the practice apparently continues to be both strategic and binding. And while very different in origin from Muslim milk siblingship, breast milk sharing in the American context is also a thoroughly modern affair.

After Anuka's first donation we kept in touch with photos and emails about our kids' development. When our son turned one, she wrote us a lovely letter wishing him a happy birthday and asked if she could send him hand-me-downs (which we naturally said we would love to receive). When she decided briefly to return to Cairo during the Arab Spring we periodically touched base with her to make sure she was safe. We continued to stay in touch and spent the day together when she and her children visited us in the fall of 2016.

I knew that this would probably be a unique experience. I live in Savannah, Georgia, where the population is not especially diverse. There are few Muslims here, and I did not expect to have many, or any, other donors who would offer milk siblingship. And while this expectation was borne out, others were not. I expected, for example, that most of the women involved in the group (and we met more than fifty when all was said and done) would be "lefty," highly educated, Volvo-driving types. They were instead often "righty," conservative, Christian home-schoolers who were wary of government and Western medicine.

Although many health professionals warn about the dangers involved, social media–enabled, person-to-person breast milk sharing is now going global. And while there are risks in accepting and giving a child another woman's milk, many people find these risks manageable. It is likely that as more parents—those with a need for milk or those who have milk to give—become aware of milk sharing, the practice will become more common. As milk sharing expands I suspect there will be vigorous push-back from institutions such as the Human Milk Banking Association of North America (HMBANA) that may have much to lose—from money to access to human milk donations for research to a sense of authority—by the mainstreaming of milk sharing. I must agree with Akre, Gribble, and Minchin (2011), who suggest that people involved in milk sharing are likely be undeterred by unsupportive or even critical public health voices; I suspect that donors will continue to provide breast milk to those who prefer to nourish their children with human milk rather than formula.

Having weaned my own kids, I turned my energies to exploring more systematically what these exchanges might suggest about the larger political, economic, and cultural contexts in which they take place. Anthropologists are tasked with the study of powerful but hard-to-see structures, such as policy, ideology, or even design conventions. I had stumbled upon what seemed a relatively invisible phenomenon, but I have since discovered that there are quite a few of us, using various methodologies and different theoretical lenses, working to understand what milk sharing is and what we can learn from it. I am convinced that studying milk sharing will provide many interesting revelations.

Acknowledgments

Producing this book has been an experience in the best sense of the term, but it would not have been even remotely possible without the help of many people and organizations. I can never adequately express my gratitude to all of the mothers (and fathers) who shared milk and their stories with me. I also want to thank the Wenner-Gren Foundation; a Wenner-Gren Hunt Post-Doctoral Fellowship was absolutely essential to the completion of this project. This project was also supported by a stipend from the Savannah College of Art and Design faculty awards program. I would like to thank Beth Concepcion, dean of the School of Liberal Arts, for providing crucial advice and support.

All of my work seems to circle around a set of questions about meaning and agency. I must acknowledge the awesome Richard Smythe and McLean Brice for helping me to hone strategies for exploring these issues early on. Initial work on breast milk sharing was presented in conference panels. Julian Brash, Jeff Mascovsky, Elsa Davidson, Elana Shever, Kristin Lawler, and Genese Sodikoff heard various iterations of this research, and I thank them for their feedback (and forbearance) and encouragement as I worked through my ideas.

I would also like to thank the many students, friends, mentors, and colleagues who talked with me about this project, read all or part of this manuscript, and gave me their honest assessment. Vincent Crapanzano, Lisa Young, Nancy Abelmann, Jayne Howell, Penny Van Esterik, Peter Biella, Catherine Kingfisher, Paul Stoller, Stephanie Takaragawa, Kate Newell, Scott Singheisen, David Stivers, Mary Doll, Larisa Honey, Steven Cox, Andrea Morrell, Julie Rogers-Varland, Allison Jablonko, Jerome Crowder, Thomas Blakely, Jonathan Marion, Liz Sargent, Capri Rosenberg, Tracy Cox-Stanton (and her cards), Sheila Matyjasik Edwards,

Jessica Smith, and Jean Murley in particular kept me from going off the rails. My father, Gene Falls, reads and responds to every last word of my work—possibly the only one to do so—and has listened thoughtfully to the (good, and bad!) ideas leading up to this book.

A special acknowledgment goes to James Bielo, who encouraged me to pursue a manuscript on this topic. James Bielo as well as Derek Krissof, Carrie Lane, and Alicia Christianson at the University of Nebraska Press carefully read various drafts of this work; their comments have improved it greatly. Erin Martineau, colleague and friend, did, as always, a superb job of editing the manuscript at all stages; her knowledge of anthropology and beyond improved this book immeasurably.

Two insightful external reviewers identified strengths and potential weaknesses of the text. I want to express my deep gratitude for their sensitive, close, and generous reading. I thank them for their helpful suggestions. The book is much better for their input.

White Gold was inspired by my discovery of the late architect Lebbeus Woods. I am forever indebted to Aleksandra Wagner for listening to my ideas (with her third ear), reading the manuscript, and entertaining my request to include images from the Lebbeus Woods estate. I hope that readers will be as stimulated as I am by Woods's work.

I am lucky to have a circle of people encouraging me: Tinka Falls, Anne Falls, Valerie Lee, Angie Dukes, Debbie Dukes, Darrell Dukes, Job Moore, Katherine Falls Menghedoht, Lee Falls, and Ifetayo White have helped me to turn the idea of this book into a reality. Thank you Dare, Zim, and Tallulah. Nothing would be possible without you.

Abbreviations

AAP	American Academy of Pediatrics
ACA	Affordable Care Act
BMS	breast milk sharing (also breast milk substitute)
CF	cystic fibrosis
CMV	cytomegalovirus
DES	diethylstilbestrol
EBF	exclusive breastfeeding
EBM	expressed breast milk
EOF	Eats on Feets
FB	Facebook
FTT	failure to thrive
HMBANA	Human Milk Banking Association of North America
HM4HB	Human Milk for Human Babies
HMF	human milk fortifier
ILCA	International Lactation Consultant Association
LLL	La Leche League International
NEC	necrotizing enterocolitis
NICU	neonatal intensive care unit
OT	occupational therapy
OTB	Only The Breast
PM	personal message
POP	persistent organic pollutant
PDHM	pasteurized donor human milk
PPACA	Patient Protection and Affordable Care Act
PPD	postpartum depression
SAHM	stay-at-home mom
SI	Situationist International

SNS   supplemental nursing system
TMJ   temporomandibular joint dysfunction
WIC   Special Supplemental Nutrition Program for Women, Infants,
       and Children

White Gold

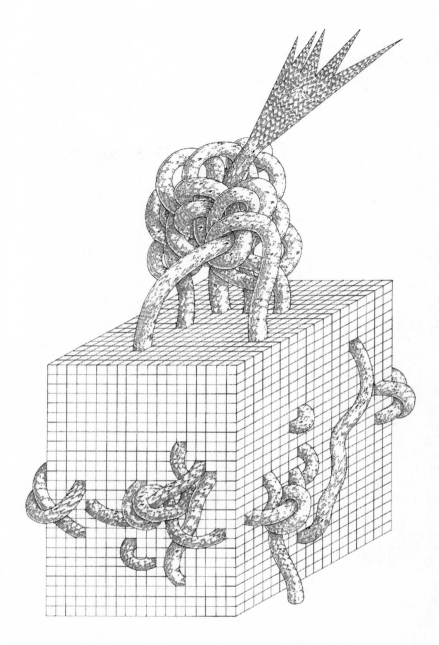

1. Lebbeus Woods, architect, American (1940–2012), *Untitled (Lost and Found 5)*, 1973. Ink on paper, 10 × 16 inches. © Estate of Lebbeus Woods.

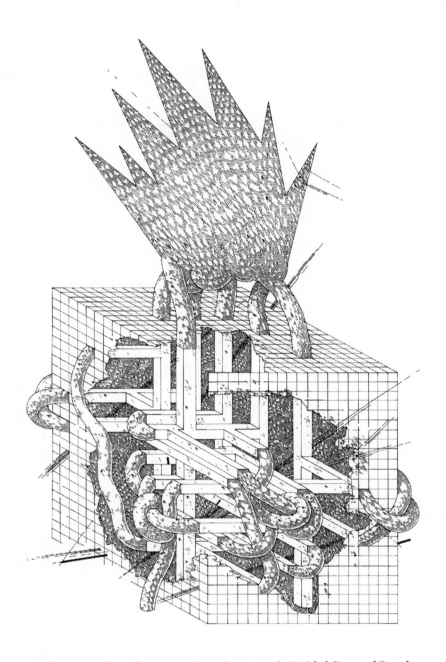

2. Lebbeus Woods, architect, American (1940–2012), *Untitled (Lost and Found 6)*, 1973. Ink on paper, 10 × 16 inches. © Estate of Lebbeus Woods. Woods was a consummate thinker and draftsman. Present in these early drawings are ideational threads—conflict and transformation—that characterize his subsequent work.

Introduction

WHITE GOLD

Women have been feeding babies at the breast for all of human history, although the particulars of feeding have varied across time and space regarding who fed the baby, when the baby was fed, when the baby was weaned, and when and what additional food was offered. In the United States fewer and fewer women breastfed their children following the introduction of synthetic milk, or "formula," during the early twentieth century. As formula came to be seen as more convenient, more modern, and even better than human milk, breastfeeding continued to fall out of fashion until advocates and health officials started pushing for a reintroduction of breastfeeding during the last quarter of the century.

The powerful "breast milk is best" campaign advanced by the American Academy of Pediatrics (AAP) and La Leche League International (LLL) tells us that breast milk is superior to formula and by extension that making milk is a shining emblem of successful motherhood. However, many mothers find, to their own frustration if not sadness or shame, that they cannot produce milk or that they cannot produce enough. Adoptive parents, surrogate parents, grandparents, and foster parents may also want to provide breast milk to their children but cannot themselves produce it. And if you can't make it yourself, there are very few options. Wet nurses are hard to find nowadays. You can purchase milk from a milk bank, but it requires a prescription and is very expensive. And unless your baby is born prematurely, meets the "very low birth weight" criterion, and/or is in a neonatal intensive care unit (NICU), it is almost impossible to access banked milk. The alternative? Acquire breast milk through direct, "peer-to-peer" exchange.

White Gold is an anthropological account of a breast milk sharing network in the southern United States. Contemporary forms of capitalism, motherhood, community, and risk reflect each other in this emerg-

3

ing practice that connects donors and recipients through digital social media. My research was partly autobiographical because of my own involvement with the network, but that was only the starting point. The center of this account is grounded in narratives gathered through formal interviews with donors, doulas, medical professionals, and other donees. I have worked to couch sharers' stories within work by anthropologists who have studied breast milk from many angles, for example, as a biological (Sellen 2012) or biocultural substance (Fouts, Hewlett, and Lamb 2012; Van Esterik 1992, 2006), as a mode of feeding in developing countries (Van Esterik 1989; Van Hollen 2011; Kroeker and Beckwith 2011), as a medium for kinship (El Guindi 2011, 2012; Altorki 1980), as a nexus for negotiating gender (Gottschang 2007), as an index of environmental dynamics (Farmer 1988), and so forth. There is also a small but quickly expanding body of work by Beatriz Reyes-Foster, Aunchalee Palmquist, Katherine Carroll, and Tanya Cassidy, who use questionnaires, discourse analysis, and quantitative and qualitative methods to examine milk bank donation and informal sharing. *White Gold* adds to these studies in cleaving breast milk from breastfeeding to look at the meanings of shared milk as it is circulated and consumed, doing so through a regional ethnographic study launched from my own point of view.

Breast milk is conceptualized by sharers as "white gold"—a scarce, valuable, and even magical substance. This book shows that sharing it is a mode of enacting parenthood, cultural values, and care, all via a dynamic, decentered network. It is a fascinating example of need-based community making between strangers in the context of contemporary commodity capitalism. I have examined this phenomenon using several anthropological lenses, starting with kinship but then turning to exchange, agency, and infrastructure. This sequence made sense to me because mothers' milk is being commodified at a very rapid clip.

Sharing

In my experience people are surprised to hear that strangers are sharing milk and that it is free. I myself recall being a little shocked to learn that doing so was even possible. Even after we started sharing, a friend confessed to me, "Now I'm used to it, but in the beginning it freaked me out to see all of those bags of milk in your fridge." Claudia, another friend I interviewed, recalled how it seemed rather suspicious at first: "You know, the first time I heard about [sharing] from April, she was explaining to me how they did it—you know, how they did the exchange—and I thought it sounded like a drug run in the middle of the night. You know, 'meet me on the bridge at 1:30 for the pickup'!" And frankly it does take on an underground, somewhat clandestine tang when described in those terms.

Since the practice is not well known, I first describe the basics of how milk is shared. And since this project is somewhat unusual in that I began the study from my own experience, I dedicate some time to explaining my research methods. I have many roles: wife, mother, sister, daughter, friend, and teacher, but I am also an anthropologist, whether I'm at the hardware store or a birthday party, in a swimming pool or reading blogs on the Internet. Given this identity, I was automatically positioned as a participant-observer within the sharing network, and several things both surprised and excited the anthropologist in me right from the get-go. And while I had no plans to write about milk sharing at first, when my youngest child transitioned off of milk I found myself thinking about all the women I had met and how these sharing relationships were embedded in the world. Over time I began to see sharing as a refusal to abdicate competency to institutionalized authority. But I am getting way ahead of myself. Let me back up and start with the basic matter of feeding babies.

Promising Evidence

What is the best source of nutrition for babies? Americans hear in the media and from doctors that breast milk is best, but is there really a meaningful difference between breastfeeding and formula feeding? Is formula bad for us? Are brands of formula significantly different from one another? To answer these questions I, like many other parents, had done some sleuthing on the Internet. A mountain of materials advanced the "breast is best" narrative, but some, such as "The Case against Breast-Feeding" in the *Atlantic*, questioned whether the pressure to breastfeed was more helpful than harmful given some of the "murky correlations" between breastfeeding and long-term health (Rosin 2009). More recently a *New York Times* article, "Overselling Breastfeeding" (Jung 2015), bemoaned the "righteous zeal" expressed by advocates against the fact that studies show only a modest benefit. Like others I spoke with, I found all of the information confusing: I concluded that there was promising evidence but not absolute proof that breast milk was better than formula for infant health but also that formula would not harm children.

So I was open to formula in principle. I thought, "Heck, I was raised on formula! And I seem to be okay." Frankly until having my own children I never gave the milk versus formula debate a single thought. But given a choice I preferred to give breast milk to my own babies. After all, like other Americans, I had been told by doctors, lactation consultants, family members, and other mothers that breast milk is better than formula, and I had sensed the underlying implication that good motherhood is synonymous with breastfeeding. Rhonda Shaw (2010) has argued that this marketing goes even further in portraying the breastfeeding mother as good, while those who use formula are stigmatized as noncompliant. At times I heard mothers in my own community echoing this sentiment.

Admittedly in the beginning I was not particularly critical of the "breast milk is best" idea since it just seemed logical to me that mothers' milk, which had evolved over millions of years to nourish infants, would be superior to a manufactured substitute produced by profit-seeking companies using sophisticated marketing campaigns to sell the idea of formula as superior. Companies have managed to insert themselves into hospital swag bags: materials given to new mothers often contain coupons for or samples of formula.

We gave our son hospital-provided formula when he was born. It turned out that he had an allergic reaction to the first product, which had cow's milk as a base. A hospital pediatrician then suggested we try a soy-based variety once we got home. But when I read the ingredients on the labels of several brand-name formulas, I thought, *I wouldn't drink that, why would I ask my baby to?* Take a look at the list of ingredients in Similac's Go & Grow Soy-Based Early Shield Powder:

Corn Syrup (38%), Soy Protein Isolate (16%), High Oleic Safflower Oil (11%), Sugar (10%), Soy Oil (8%), Coconut Oil (7%), Calcium Phosphate (3%). Less than 2% of the following: C. Cohnii Oil, M. Alpina Oil, Beta-Carotene, Lutein, Lycopene, Fructooligosaccharides,

Potassium Citrate, Salt, Magnesium Chloride, Ascorbic Acid, L-Methionine, Potassium Chloride, Choline Chloride, Taurine, Ferrous Sulfate, Ascorbyl Palmitate, m-Inositol, Mixed Tocopherols, Zinc Sulfate, d-Alpha-tocopheryl Acetate, L-Carnitine, Niacinamide, Calcium Carbonate, Calcium Pantothenate, Cupric Sulfate, Thiamine Chloride Hydrochloride, Vitamin A Palmitate, Riboflavin, Pyridoxine Hydrochloride, Folic Acid, Potassium Iodide, Phylloquinone, Biotin, Vitamin D3, Cyanocobalamin, Sodium Selenate, and Potassium Hydroxide.

Now, breast milk does taste sweet, but I was taken aback when I saw this list, and I was not at all thrilled with the idea of giving a baby something that was made with 38 percent corn syrup. But because almost everyone assumed that we, as adoptive parents, would use formula, the only real question was what brand, so we tried to find one that had less corn syrup. It was only when I encountered the midwife-doula-"lactivist" circuit that I learned of any alternatives.

Several doulas suggested that I could try to induce breast milk production using a combination of hormone therapy and pumping. Every mother has different goals and needs, and this treatment was more than I was willing to try, but I also learned much to my surprise that some men were also attempting this, so great was their desire to breastfeed. I learned from Jared Diamond (1995) that anthropologists have "known for some time that many male mammals, including some men, can undergo breast development and lactate under special conditions."

I also discovered that when milk induction is unsuccessful or milk production is inadequate, parents will sometimes feed an infant formula or breast milk through a small tube taped to the breast using a simulated nursing system, with the idea that this activity will encourage both bonding and lactation. After seeing my friends and sister breastfeed their children, I could certainly understand the desire to connect with a child in this way. I was drawn to the possibility of celebrating the togetherness that comes from feeding and to the idea of using breast milk for food. And so that is just what we did, through milk sharing. Once we started looking, we were able to feed our children donated milk, all obtained via the sharing group, without supplementing with formula.

Not everyone can breastfeed or chooses to breastfeed or use donated milk, and formula is a convenient, workable alternative or, as Joan Wolf describes it, a "remarkable example of human ingenuity" (2013, 150). I fully recognize that breastfeeding makes substantial demands on mothers' time, psyche, and energy, and I have no interest in questioning or criticizing those who make the choice to use formula either some or all of the time. So while I do track the outlines of the "breast is best" campaign as it relates to sharing, I do not directly enter into ongoing disputes— scientific, moral, or otherwise—about the value of formula versus breastfeeding. The women and men that I interacted with and interviewed, for the most part, took it as a given that, if and when possible, infants should consume human milk rather than formula. As a mother I felt the same way, but I also wondered about the source of this preference. To explore, I could not help but to activate my identity as an anthropologist. I found myself doing ethnography at home in the most literal of ways.

Anthropology at Home

Following the critiques of "armchair" anthropology by both W. H. R. Rivers (1913) and Bronislaw Malinowski ([1922] 1984), researchers stopped relying on travelers' notebooks and began conducting fieldwork themselves, staying in the field for extended periods of time, learning local languages, taking copious notes on both everyday and extraordinary events, and, in accordance with Malinowski's mandate, "putting aside camera, note book and pencil, to join in himself in what is going on. He can take part in the natives' games, he can follow them on their visits and walks, sit down and listen and share in their conversations" ([1922] 1984, 21). Doing so would help one "to grasp the native's point of view, his relation to life, to realize *his* vision of *his* world," Malinowski adds (25).

These new guidelines produced different kinds of materials. You would note upon reading reflections on fieldwork by both Rivers and Malinowski an assumption that the ethnographer is working among "savages" or "natives" and living at a distance from the metropole, geographically, culturally, and otherwise. Anthropological studies in the early twentieth century were undertaken in foreign locales with people who were considered, if not exotic, then at least "other." It would be decades before many anthropologists would specialize in Western societies, even though early founders of the field, such as Margaret Mead and Franz Boas, promoted the study of American society as not only a worthwhile but also an imperative endeavor.

Many late nineteenth- and early twentieth-century anthropologists working in the United States focused on Native American populations, sometimes in the form of critiques of governmental policy. Others conducted research with African Americans, white urbanites, and ethnic minorities. These studies continue to shape the central concerns of anthropological research in the United States.

Some midcentury work would become classic: W. Lloyd Warner's (1941) work on Yankee City provided a model for work on race, class, industrial relations, and local politics in complex urban centers. Other work was simply ahead of its time. Hortense Powdermaker (1950), for example, conducted an innovative study of Hollywood's film industry, a topic that would have raised eyebrows well into the 1990s. And while what Powdermaker and contemporaries such as Zora Neale Hurston and Melville Herskovits were doing was not called "anthropology at home," that's exactly what it was (see Peirano 1998). Other terms created to describe conducting anthropological research in one's own society include "native ethnography," "indigenous anthropology," "introspective research," and so forth.

These neologisms struggle to describe something that differs from traditional studies of foreign colonial or postcolonial others, and they point to a disciplinary state of affairs in which anthropologists have had to justify the United States as an area of investigation. And while many scholars now conduct fieldwork "at home" (especially after they have proven their chops working abroad), it is instructive to note that the Society for the Anthropology of North America, now a mid-sized section of the larger American Anthropological Association, was founded in the early 1980s by Ida Susser and Maria Vesperi.

Today anthropologists examining life in the United States work in urban centers and suburban neighborhoods, as well in small rural communities, at a wide range of sites and with all kinds of people; park designers, grassroots organizers, galleristas, animal sanctuary workers, nongovernmental organization officers, corporate managers, scientists, and tour guides are just a few examples. A great deal of this work focuses

on issues related to race, class, gender, sexuality, nationality, and eth-
nicity, but others study immigration, education, militarization, the
prison-industrial complex, deindustrialization, indigeneity, social movements, disability studies, the New Right, science and technology, labor,
the arts, food and the body, and more. As Ida Susser (2001) has pointed
out, as global interrelationships and the glaring inequalities that accompany them intensify, studying American society and power will continue
to have major ramifications for our understandings of events and experiences in other national contexts.

Complicating the notion of doing anthropology at home today is the
fact that people are moving around like never before. The rise of mul-
ticulturalism and identity politics in this context can make the categories
of "home" and "abroad" redundant, irrelevant, or even confusing: just
where does an Indian-American immigrant living in Buenos Aires do
"anthropology at home"? Are anthropological studies of virtual communities "at home"? Does doing anthropology at home imply studying
a giant imagined national community? Or does "home" more accurately
describe a subculture? What is home, exactly?

Taking the notion of "at home" literally, the authors of *Life at Home
in the Twenty-First Century* (Arnold et al. 2012) use a combination archae-
ological and material culture approach to explore middle-class consum-
erism in Los Angeles, while David Halle's *Inside Culture: Art and Class
in the American Home* (1994) examines how people exhibit and interpret
aesthetic objects. Both books draw fascinating conclusions about contemporary American life, which the authors gleaned by interviewing
residents and documenting their interior living spaces, but neither book
depicts the homes of the author or authors. These studies at home, in
homes, are excellent examples of how images can be used in life and in
ethnographic texts but are not particularly reflexive in terms of exploring the intimate lives of authors.

Since scholars started calling attention to issues of identity, positionality,
partiality, and power inherent in the act of (mostly first-world elites) representing others (particularly colonial, postcolonial, or minority others),
anthropologists have struggled to find new ways to become more reflexive
(Asad 1973). This means taking stock of the ways in which one's own nationality, race, class, gender, sexuality, or even personality may impact field site

selection, experience, and analysis. Being explicit about one's own identity contextualizes and can even strengthen the arguments one makes.

So how are field sites typically selected? In the United States graduate students are encouraged to study abroad so that they will learn how to navigate a radically "other" milieu. Some anthropologists even argue that you must do ethnographic work abroad if you are to be a *real* anthropologist, because only then are you sufficiently equipped to do work in the United States. Even when studying centers of global capital junior researchers may confront the perception that doing research "at home" does not sufficiently train them to negotiate cultural difference and to reevaluate ethnocentric and atheoretical approaches to society (Susser 2001, 7–8). But Susser points out that crossing class boundaries, for example, can lead to cultural dissonance as challenging and illuminating as crossing national or ethnic boundaries (8). I would add that encountering other styles, values, or aesthetic preferences can have a similarly illuminating effect. Even taking the self as a subject of ethnographic study can be productive in this sense.

Moving about as far away as you can get from studying a foreign, exotic other is the practice of undertaking research on your own community, with yourself as the primary informant, as Kathleen Stewart and Randol Contreras have done. Stewart's *Ordinary Affects* (2008) tracks the identity, observations, and everyday experiences of the author through a series of (rather poetic) vignettes. The entire text can be read as an exercise in phenomenological anthropology and as a commentary on the politics of race, class, and gender under the conditions of globalized neoliberal governmentality.

While Stewart presents herself in the third person, Contreras tells a first-person version of his life growing up in the South Bronx in *The Stickup Kids: Race, Violence, and the American Dream* (2012). In his account of "gangsta' life" Contreras helpfully addresses his own struggle with issues of objectivity; he had to debate, for example, what to tell and what to hold back, imagining how his friends might feel about how he was telling their stories. He also had to consider how his tenure committee might reframe their understanding of a colleague who they would now discover had participated in a life of crime.

I have tried to learn from these examples how to remain both true to and critically aware of my own subject position as a relatively well off, educated white woman, born and raised in the South, who has lived a substantial portion of my adult life exploring the lives and practices of people in other places. My identity in this project, postmodern as this may sound, is one of multiple perspectives. I could not help but to tack back and forth between being a mother and an anthropologist as I made new friends and learned the ropes of breast milk sharing.

Biases inevitably pervade the material I collected, but having initially participated in sharing as a donee allowed me to understand what's at stake, perhaps even better than someone discovering this practice more "objectively," from the outside. My perspectives as a mother and as an anthropologist are complementary (see Chang 2008; Ellis and Bochner 2000): as a mother, I experienced an affective understanding of the various potencies of milk sharing that might have otherwise remained obscured (see Jones 2005; Cassidy 2012), and, as an anthropologist, I was attuned to theory playing in the everyday.

Augmenting my efforts to account for my own subject position was my reading about autoethnography (Kelley and Betsalel 2004; Ellis 2004; Hayano 1979; Maréchal 2010; Hunt and Junco 2006). I have attempted to avoid presenting work that is overly subjective by satisfying conditions defined by Anderson (2006, 373): autoethnographers should be a "complete member of the social world under study," engage reflectively on themselves, be visibly and actively present in the text, include other informants in similar situations, and be committed to theoretical analysis. Thus, the evidence marshaled for this book is a combination of autoethnographic study with established techniques of investigation such as interviewing, analyzing documents, historical research, and contextualization (Buzard 2003; Ellingson and Ellis 2008; Reed-Danahay 1997). I was especially energized by Heewon Chang's *Autoethnography as Method* (2008), which provides step-by-step guidelines for mining experience and reinforced my own impulses to avoid an excessive focus on myself. So while I have developed theoretical explanations of social phenomena from my own experience, mine is not the only voice, nor is it the focus of this work (Ellington and Ellis 2008, 445; see also Denzin and Lincoln 1994; Ellis 2004; and Sparkes 2000). My work on *White Gold* extends well beyond my own involvement through interviews I conducted with donees, husbands, doulas, lactation consultants, medical professionals, and donors. I can only hope that I struck a decent balance.

Finding the Subject in Self and Substance

Joslyn was a far more typical donor than Anuka (the Egyptian architect described in the preface). She is culturally conservative. Her working-class husband is in law enforcement. Joslyn cared for their three boys, making cloth diapers and attending an evangelical church, sometimes dropping off her donation on her way to a part-time job at a children's clothing shop at the mall. We found ways to give Joslyn tokens of appreciation, such as Christmas tree ornaments or a pair of grab-proof earrings. When I went to her house, she usually invited me to sit down and offered me a beverage. Sometimes we put the babies down on the floor and let them look at each other and laugh. We talked about parenting or our babies' new skills. The exchange was often a social occasion, although there were times that I simply picked up bags of milk, threw them in a cooler with a hunk of dry ice, and drove away—sometimes feeling a little like something was missing and sometimes not.

All told, we had well more than fifty donors. I was fascinated by the stories that people were telling me, and I had kept notes all along, but when we began breast milk sharing with our second child and I was (slightly) less overwhelmed, I began looking at sharing from a different, decidedly more anthropological, perspective. I read oft-cited work related to milk, such as *Mothers and Medicine* (Apple 1987), *The Anthropology of Breast-feeding* (Maher 1992), and *Giving Breastmilk* (Shaw and Bartlett 2010). Each of these works in its own way examines the practice of breastfeeding as intertwined with constructions of nature, gender, and appropriate mothering. I also explored lesser-known materials; my reading of *Banking on the Body* (2014) by the legal scholar Kara Swanson not only helped me understand the early history of milk banking but also provided a lawyerly take on commodification, especially with regard to the delineation between private versus civic property.

Asef Bayat's (2000, 2010) work on ordinary people's responses to the crush of neoliberal governance in the Middle East helped me to think about milk sharing as a form of agency. The comments that informants made during formal interviews led me to still other texts, and I followed those leads, albeit in a rather creative, perhaps somewhat idiosyncratic way. Doing so took me to biological and medical research on milk itself (of which there is a great deal), popular press on contemporary forms of milk sharing (of which there is little), and articles on the phenomenal growth of the for-profit human milk industry.

In the end I conducted formal interviews with more than forty participants who were involved in breast milk sharing (a few were our donors, but most were not). I focused on donors and donees, but I also talked with doulas, nurses, and doctors, many of whom I located using a snowball technique. Since most informants either knew me or knew of me through the local network, I was in an excellent position to pose a loose set of questions that allowed them to talk about their experiences, motivations, and broader life histories. I allowed people a great deal of latitude to discuss how and why they become involved, as well as to comment on their expectations, hopes, and disappointments. I did not directly ask about political affiliations or economic standing but allowed these to emerge obliquely. I explained to participants that the intention of my study was to learn more about how milk sharing was practiced as part of my research for a book I was writing, and I took handwritten notes during interviews (largely editing out "ums" and "ahs"). I remained as true as I could to informants' voices, both in my fieldnotes and in this book, but in order to protect the privacy of participants I followed the standard ethnographic practice of changing names and identifying details. I have also taken the liberty of combining or splitting identities where necessary to protect privacy.

Issues of class and race figure prominently in studies of breastfeeding and indeed in my own sharing experience. As Avishai (2011) points out, even though the percentages of mothers breastfeeding had rebounded to 70 percent by the mid-2000s in response to the push by the American Academy of Pediatrics, it is hardly surprising, given that breastfeeding requires access to resources, nourishment, and a relaxing (and possibly private) environment, that white, middle-class, educated, heterosexually paired, older mothers who stay at home are much more likely than other women to initiate breastfeeding, to continue beyond the first few days, and to keep feeding their children breast milk when and if they return to work.

Echoing this statistic, the vast majority our donors, and the donors and donees I interviewed, were like Joslyn: middle-class, married, white mothers. Many had graduated from college or had some college-level education, but there were a few who had not had any college coursework and others who had postgraduate degrees. Many donors were stay-at-home moms living in detached houses, with husbands who worked as police officers, small business owners, sales agents, real-estate agents, professors, managers, lawyers, and so forth. There are several large military bases nearby, and several husbands worked for the military. Some donors were themselves enlisted. Women who worked either before or after giving birth were employed as school counselors, retail sales clerks, schoolteachers, personal trainers, doctors, architects, farmers, and so forth, though a few worked directly with women as doulas or midwives.

After completing the interviews I coded my notes to manage them with greater ease. Interviews are odd social interactions. People are indexing (or pointing to) who they are and who they think the interviewer is, performing identities threaded with ideas about aesthetics, race, and class, and creating or disarticulating a power-rife relationship with the interviewer (Crapanzano 1985). My process of coding was therefore sensitive to the indexical properties of interviews when I could determine that these dynamics were at play. Coding also helped alleviate biases that inevitably pervaded my own autobiographical material, which resulted from having participated initially as an extremely naïve new parent. Some of the most salient variables that emerged included instinct, modernity, community, risk, mothering, altruism, gender, and medical expertise. The same practice was applied to the academic literature I studied, as well as to material obtained via social media. I focused on the website MilkShare and state-specific Facebook sites in my own region (Georgia, North Carolina, South Carolina, and Florida), looking for both conformity and outliers. This focus allowed me to locate overlaps within different levels of discourse (personal, academic, and popular).

Mine is not a quantitative study based on a large-scale questionnaire but rather an interpretive analysis of qualitative research. Data collected in interviews are not representative, nor have I used the data with the intention of enumerating frequencies or making statistical claims (Yin 1989). Instead the data were taken as a pool of narratives. Studying these narratives helped me to draw conclusions about communal responses to social and political forces, in the context of capitalism, that are taking place via the use of social media technology. I recognize moreover that parents involved with milk sharing represent a small minority (some researchers estimate that less that 1 percent of women who express milk share with another family [Stevens and Keim 2015]) and that my study is regional—conditions that impinge upon the generalizability of my findings. Further research will be needed to reveal how the findings about my own network can be applied elsewhere.

Organizing the Body Politic

This book could have been put together in a number of different ways because asking what breast milk sharing *is*, as a first step, leads to a several intriguing pathways. I could open, for example, with the nature of milk itself, the management of risk, ideas about childrearing and parenthood, the aversion to the abject, or how milk sharing resists authoritative institutions that are opposed to it. Milk sharing can be treated as a network, as a kinship practice, as dissent, as a form of biocapitalism, as affective labor, as cyborgian, as a heterarchy, as a show of agency, or as a thrilling performance of trust. As a profoundly historical contingency—unimaginable in its current form without the rise of digital technology, consumer capitalism, road and postal setups, risk society, modernity, biopolitics, and so forth—milk sharing is all of these things and none alone.

Breast milk thus presents a semiotic problem. What is milk? What is milk sharing? In following Charles Sanders Peirce's (1931–58, 2:228) dictum that a sign is something that means something to somebody, I have tried to tease apart what milk sharing "means" from various points of view. Taking what Jules David Prown (2001, 235–37) calls a "hard" approach, or seeking systematic information about the "reality of the object itself," I can examine milk, for example, through the lens of anthropology's sister sciences, such as biology, physiology, and chemistry. Conversely a "soft" approach would focus on milk's cultural and symbolic dimensions, "as part of a language through which culture speaks its mind" (Prown 2001, 237). Milk's special and mundane physical qualities (from sugar content to antibody load) are made visible using a hard approach, while a soft approach shows milk articulating ideas about nutrition, motherhood, nature, and so forth.

As I have shown in my work on diamonds (Falls 2008), milk can be understood as a duality: it is both cultural material and material culture. We can cleave the idea or concept of breast milk as cultural material from any particular example of it as material culture. What I have found useful in doing this is what Charles Sanders Peirce called a type/token distinction (Peirce 1931–58, 4:537). Types have "a definite identity, though usually admitting a great variety of appearances" (8:334). The identity of breast milk as type, for example, might be associated with how it is produced, what is in it, and its range of colors (including white, blue, or orange) and textures (viscous or thin). We might think of the type as cultural material.

Any specific instance of breast milk is a token, an exemplification of the type. Here it is material culture. We expect tokens to share some, maybe most, but not necessarily all of the qualities identified within the type "breast milk." And while types and tokens have different ontological registers, they are intimately related. Recognizing the type as abstract category and the token as a material instantiation can help us track breast milk as an agent in world-making (a point to which I return).

The type/token (or cultural material/material culture) lens allows us (indeed tells us) to take instances of breast milk as historically sited, as events that emerge and occur in time and space, refracting cultural, political, and economic dynamics. The type to which a token is attached does its work in what Law (2009) calls "mattering," in a different register. This lens encourages us to attend to historical and cultural circumstances that make milk look to us in a particular way. Then we can focus on what milk means and what it does.

Within this framework breast milk becomes understood as complicated cultural material or material culture that is entangled with patterns of circulation, agency, political economy, technology, and risk. One way to begin analyzing breast milk in this way is to recognize that it materializes or becomes an object between people, and in this sense it is relational. The mother::child dyad is one site of emergence, but milk also materializes within partnerships by people who define its use, meaning, and efficacy for other kinds of activities that may or may not align with "best practices" promoted by institutional authorities.

Constructed by sharers as "white gold," milk as a type operates as a natural foil to chemical formulas that simulate women's bodily fluid under the profit logic of capitalism. Milk as token, however, is personal, temporal, and situated. The circulation of milk, its pathway, depends upon intersecting political, economic, and cultural configurations, such as laws governing bodily fluids, commodification pushing against donor networks, and values promoted by the natural birth community. Technology—from milk-pumping-and-storing tools, to social media sites, to pharmaceuticals and drug tests, to scientific and medical practice—also shapes milk sharing.

As sharing has grown in popularity, milk has materialized as a fundable object of scientific investigation. Resulting scientific knowledge is of course then implicated in the production, maintenance, and contestation of social practices. In the scientific community milk sharing might be (and often is) viewed as "too risky" (Akre 2011). Interestingly, as milk sharing became more visible in my area between 2010 and 2014 (the same period in which scientific interest was growing), I noticed that more donors and donees were willing to, or wanted to participate in, shares that bioscience would almost certainly view as unsafe—meaning that, for example, donors did not disclose documentation regarding their HIV status and donees accepted milk from donors "no questions asked." My research traces how the relational, circulatory, and technological aspects of sharing are mobilized by participants to negotiate perceptions of risk. Mothers I spoke with appealed to forms of decision making that lie outside the parameters of rational scientific methods (which are always incomplete) to guide choices about whom to donate to or accept milk from: these forms of knowledge included instinct, women's work, group consciousness, and feelings of trust.

But what does all of this have to do with the notion of agency or world-making, as mentioned above? The issue of agency is important in anthropology because, among other things, it is future oriented. People can have agency, and the kind of agency people express has implications for progressive social action, for notions of responsibility, for consciousness. Within anthropology there has been a notable discussion about the agency of things. As a thing, milk certainly does things. It is matter that can matter. As an event, breast milk is a magnetic hub for strangers who might not and probably would not otherwise have ever come together to practice trusting one other. This stranger convergence constitutes collaborative world-making.

Knowing the history of ideas and attitudes about milk is important, but I am interested in a more pragmatic question: How and why do tokens of "liquid gold" matter? And how do they affect participants? For example, donating allows lactating women to perform an identity as a community member. By receiving milk, donees can perform a style of parenting. Values are expressed, refined, and negotiated during the talk that surrounds the exchange. For example, I saw sharers negotiating a "we-them" critique of medical and pharmaceutical policy, as reflected in one donor's description of the profit-driven formula industry: "they don't have *our* best interests at heart."

We intend ourselves into the world through material culture. We can't even imagine existing without it. So while breast milk as a type has a history (or histories) within which some core aspects of its identity are fairly persistent, owing to the fact that it is a fluid emitted from a biological organism, tokens of shared milk must be understood in their own (and usually short-lived) trajectory, with a finer level of detail, embedded in and contributing to a body politic. This is where an ethnographic approach is useful.

Ethno-graphing

So with an eye toward presenting an analysis of a relatively underresearched globalized practice from a local and somewhat personal standpoint, I begin *White Gold* with an overview of sharing. Subsequent chapters highlight different aspects of the practice: Who is involved? What are their motivations? I thus explore how milk moves, what it does, and what we can learn by looking at it ethnographically.

As a more poetic counterpoint to this fairly straightforward organization, Apollonian in its linear and disciplined argumentation, I have inserted a series of images that operate like the dithyramb sung by the chorus in a Greek tragedy. (A dithyramb works as an ode to Dionysus, meant to offer background, insight, and commentary to the main narrative but in a style that is adventurous, disorderly, poetic, and evocative.) These visual vignettes are not meant to stand alone as a parallel interbook, nor are they to be read as literal illustrations of material presented in neighboring chapters. They are bridges between the chapters and between what is said and what is not said. They are like dreams between days. They are meant to offer provocations for thinking about what milk and milk sharing are, have been, and indeed can be.

The placement of images between each chapter is different from the ethnographic exposition some readers may have learned to expect. Most anthropological books that do contain images (often photographs taken during the course of fieldwork) use them in a supporting role, as straightforward illustrations of people, places, or objects. But there are other ways that images can be used. Images created by authors or curated from art history, cinema studies, design handbooks, or even found footage can be placed to challenge, juxtapose, or even contradict prose in ways that intensify our engagement with it. Even the seeming non sequitur that presents an interpretive challenge can add an additional layer of interpretation to expository text. There is a long literary, artistic, and cinematic tradition of using visuals in what we might call purposeful interruption. I found Scott McCloud's *Understanding Comics* (1994), Michael Taussig's *I Swear I Saw This* (2011), John Steinbeck's *Grapes of Wrath* (1939), Todd Haynes's film *Poison* (1991), and Ernest Hemingway's *In Our Time* (1930) to be especially helpful in understanding how the use of images or collage can work in counterpoint.

Ethnographic exposition is typically linear, and because of this quality it can flatten cultural and historical contexts (which are by their nature ambiguous, ephemeral, and contradictory). The images in *White Gold* invite the reader to engage his or her poetic self in developing a semantic ambience surrounding my more traditional style of argumentation. The images are meant to prime you to sense and to explore connections and characteristics that are not explicitly stated. While this strategy may present an unfamiliar or even uncomfortable challenge, I can only hope that the effort will be worth it.

I have provided more scaffolding for readers in the first few sets of images, but as the reading progresses I leave readers to their own devices. This strategy aligns with what I understand Roland Barthes (1973) to be up to when he identifies the *lisable*, the readerly text, that is here working in tandem with a *scriptable*, or a writerly text (a collage of images and narration). Thinking more broadly, I hope that this strategy will contribute to our collective toolkit for presenting ethnographic material.

Following the vignette entitled "Ethno-Graphics," chapter one describes how milk moves by discussing its material and medical aspects, as well as how supposed benefits and dangers of sharing intersect with trust and risk. This chapter also describes the compound infrastructure through which milk moves and around which the modern network of sharers coalesces.

One of the most unexpected features of my experience with sharers was the general trend toward political conservatism in the donor community. Many of the families were conservative and Christian, prizing stay-at-home motherhood and homeschooling. Many were suspicious of the medical system as it relates to motherhood; they had natural childbirth at home or in natural birthing centers, designed homemade diapers, promoted slowed vaccination schedules or none at all, and of course celebrated and promoted breastfeeding. I connected with mothers with whom I might not otherwise have expected to have much in common. But the meaning of the share varied a great deal from one individual to another. Focusing on donors, chapter two explores how and why people became involved, explaining how this group, with all of its internal idiosyncrasies, operates like a counterpublic or as what I call a "counternetwork."

Taking up the theme of experience and motivations, chapter three presents donee stories. Accounts by donees reflect a palimpsest of shared values, as well as unique desires and strategies. While the metaphor of the network connotes horizontality, there are important differences not only in participants' ability to "hook in" to the infrastructure of distribution but also in their ability to shape how the practice looks and works. The counternetwork that coalesces around an infrastructure of distribution and information exchange can be described therefore as "heterarchical," that is to say, as a form of social organization that is flexible and adaptive, in which relationships shift with context, and where power is contextual. Here people participate in a self-regulating whole by choosing to engage one another, but social actors besides donors and donees also contribute to the viability of milk sharing. The flexibility and adaptability of the heterarchy make it extremely effective. As we might expect in any social organization characterized by heterarchy ("which is both a structure and a condition" [Crumley 1995, 4]), people occupy different roles over time: a donor or donee may be or become a web page administrator, doula, or lactation activist and, by extension, affect breast milk as type.

In their constructions of breast milk as type, the medical community, the Food and Drug Administration (FDA), the AAP, La Leche League International, and milk banks acknowledge that there are questions about milk exchange with regard to disease, chemical or drug exposure, and contamination that have to be navigated, and they draw the conclusion that sharing is too risky. The FDA recommends against feeding babies with milk acquired through sharing. The AAP discourages the use of unscreened donors (by which they mean screened in the way that milk banks screen donors). The Canadian Pediatric Society and the AAP also recommend against using donor milk. Banks affiliated with the Human Milk Banking Association of North America take the position that the risks of using shared milk remain so great as to make it an untenable option, and they do not support it.

Even La Leche League, the organization perhaps most often associated with the promotion of breastfeeding, does not support milk sharing. When I attempted to interview Ida, my local LLL representative, about it, she explained in an email that as a representative of LLL she was happy to share information about breastfeeding but could not speak specifically to milk sharing. Making three main points, she explained that LLL "has chosen to neither condemn nor condone this practice except to say that mothers should use caution when accepting human milk donations from outside a milk bank environment," that mothers "breastfeeding babies under six months should be cautious of the priority of their own baby's needs if they intend to donate milk and may want to speak to an LLL leader about balancing those needs," and that LLL leaders should not "initiate the suggestion of an informal milk-donation arrangement or act as an intermediary in such a situation, but can only provide unbiased information about the risks and benefits of such an arrangement." She directed me to consult the LLL website if I had further questions.

As with LLL, "lactivists" promote the value of milk for infant health and development (Faircloth 2009, 2013; Lunceford 2012). Chapter four examines sharing as a form of ideologically powered community work, situated within a larger institutional context that finds milk sharing too risky. Ideas about self-sufficiency, a desire to avoid the commercialism associated with babies, a mistrust of pharmaceutical and food industries and the governmental bodies that regulate them, and the desire to promote "women's knowledge" and labor, as well as heartfelt commitments to support local communities, were motivations that lactivists described. As with other issues, activism around the politics of milk, including sharing, is diverse, taking place at many levels and with varying degrees of consciousness or strategizing: some simply participate in sharing, acting as a model that others may or may not follow in what I would call microactivism, while at the other extreme advocate-lactivists may demand that children receive breast milk no matter what, even if it means overriding a mother's wishes. I would argue that the microactivism that introduces milk sharing to the family and friends of sharers is a more private but crucial flip side to the ways in which more visible lactivists are shaping milk as type and, therefore, cultural attitudes about milk sharing (though these of course do not go uncontested).

As the benefits of milk are promoted and interest in the circulation of milk grows, milk is acquiring commercial value. Since capitalism always seeks new markets and new commodities and finds new ways to extract value from life itself, milk sharing (along with the infrastructure and counternetwork surrounding it) has been identified as an attractive frontier for entrepreneurial biocapitalism. Frictions and convergences between sharers and biocapitalists expose the political and economic tenets that structure everyday life. Focusing on the monetization of milk, chapter five examines how commercialism, kinship, and religion converge around milk sharing. There is, perhaps not surprisingly, increasing pressure to commoditize milk as the practice becomes more mainstream, and this is happening in a technologizing, political environment. Modern technologies associated with pumping, community making, body modification (changes in breast size, for example), and reproduction (such as surrogacy and in vitro fertilization) also have an impact on the intersection of capital and sharing (Griswold 2005; Steiner 2013).

A refusal to participate in the commodification of breast milk using an unregulated sharing infrastructure is a way of refusing to reduce life to capital, and I cannot help but to wonder what legal, cultural, or economic techniques might soon make informal sharing more difficult. As an emergent and rapidly changing practice, breast milk sharing has an uncertain future. What might this look like in five or ten years, or even further out? How might it align with other experimental modes of dissent?

Disciplines outside of anthropology offer different paradigms of looking, helping us to imagine what milk sharing might inform, critique, or become. To deal with these important questions, in the last chapter I draw upon the work of the late architect Lebbeus Woods to discover what milk sharing means in terms of imaginaries, strategies, and practices that shape and are shaped by future realities. Occupying what Woods calls a "free space," milk sharing is a unique informal economy formed not solely out of necessity but as a counternetwork that functions as political-economic critique, asset-based community building, and resistance, even as it unwittingly supports, or even reproduces, some of the very conditions sharers seek to disrupt.

Ultimately this book is about an evanescent, alternative practice of people responding to problems posed by social and institutional forces. Alliances between families of the Left and the Right, making an "end run" around powerful commercial industries, functioning largely through social media, represent a distinctly contemporary form of community making, one that is taking place in the throes of what Rancière (2010) calls dissensus. Milk sharing is a model for the circulation of material culture and ideas of many kinds, and it lends texture to the body politic as a surprising, empowering, and diverse form of civil society.

Meanwhile, for most people milk sharing is still relatively under the radar. My sister reminded me one day when we were talking on the phone that

> it probably does not enter most peoples' minds to do this. And a few people I know have adopted: one friend, they were maybe a little younger than us, had two open adoptions, and so they were there at the birth and everything, and they were just handed the baby and a bottle, and they never went outside of that. So, I just think that unless you have a doula or midwife who is really open-minded and knows, your pediatrician is definitely *not* going to tell you about this. Even a

forward-thinking pediatrician is going to say, "Formula!" I mean after six months, they ask you how the breastfeeding is going, and if you say "good," they encourage you to continue, but if you are having issues, they will suggest working to find an appropriate formula. I have *never* heard anyone say that their pediatrician suggested milk sharing.

While this book is unlikely to be handed out by pediatricians, some readers may hear from a friend that she is a donor or receives milk, or perhaps lactating readers may consider donating milk. I hope that *White Gold* will help people to understand and evaluate this practice for themselves.

Thinking more broadly, we need to find better ways to live together as we struggle with the increasingly serious environmental, political, and economic challenges posed by life in the Anthropocene. I am arguing here that milk sharing, as a counternetwork of strange bedfellows coalescing around an infrastructure in the context of commodity capitalism, shows us one such better way to live together. If we are to survive as a species, the knowledge and ability to successfully trust each other and feed infants without the help of institutional authorities must be maintained. Breast milk sharing is just a small piece of the solution, but this book will be a success if it inspires readers to imagine other ways of sharing in other free spaces that may exist just beyond the horizon, allowing us to practice alternative modes of exchange and community making that operate not just as an implicit critique of exiting realities but that, even more significantly, bring different people together in new ways.

Ethno-Graphics

Paul Klee pointed out that art does not reproduce the world of the visible; it *makes the world visible*. Anthropology is *artistic* in this sense. This disciplinary kinship helps explain why artists and anthropologists borrow ideas and techniques from one another. But ethnographies typically privilege text, diminishing other ways of showing. And let's face it: language does offer specificity while images evoke strong feelings and contradictory emotions. But words and images complement each other.[1] The rational and the sensory can be, in fact always are, entwined in lived experience.

With this in mind I offer a series of vignettes as inspiration for oblique engagements: I mean for them to sensitize you to themes presented in contiguous chapters and to suggest how figurations of milk reflect, critique, and comment on political, economic, technological, and even biological notions of being human. Ancient and medieval paintings, for example, project religiously endowed worldviews, while modernist works connote an emerging secular humanism, and contemporary artists explore postmodern ideas about the body, commenting on the cyborgian aspects of motherhood and milk, the dynamics of capitalism, and feminist politics.[2]

Any history—art or otherwise—is never a seamless narrative; when done well, it contains unpredictable idiosyncrasies, wrong turns, and counterstories that define the real context. As a historically contingent practice, milk sharing explains, echoes, resists, and succeeds within a larger cultural milieu.

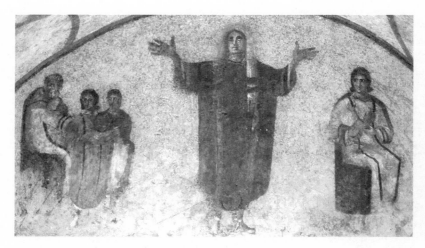

3. Detail of third-century fresco depicting Mary nursing Jesus, Catacombs of Priscilla (Rome, Italy). https://en.wikipedia.org/wiki/Catacomb_of_Priscilla#/media/File: Madonna_catacomb.jpg.

Origin Stories

Medieval and Renaissance art often featured the Virgin Mary, at times nursing the Baby Jesus. This Nursing Madonna shows up in visual culture as early as the third century. The Madonna Lactans became more common-place over the next centuries, especially with the growth of twelfth-century religious cults, which celebrated images featuring Mary's exposed breasts (Manes 2011). The façade of the Basilica di Santa Maria in Trastevere, Rome, is one such example. This mosaic, dated between the thirteenth and four-teenth centuries, was produced during a time when upper- and middle-class families hired wet nurses to breastfeed their children.

Other twelfth-century ideas operated in tension with Madonna Lac-tans imagery. Pope Innocent describes the correct medieval attitude toward humanity in his twelfth-century treatise *On the Misery of the Human Condition*: "Man was formed of dust, slime, and ashes; what is even more vile, of the filthiest seed. He was conceived from the itch of the flesh, in the heat of passion and the stench of lust, and worse yet, with the stain of sin. He was born to toil, dread and trouble; and more wretched still, was born only to die" (Lothario de Segni 1190–98).

When I asked Miranda, a milk donor who also happens to be an art historian, about these images, she remarked, "You know, in the medieval world, the body is horrid, or in the words of St. Augustine, 'a thing born between feces and urine,' and human life is miserable. So, there you would not expect to see a bodily Madonna squirting out milk." Miranda paused, "But, Enter the Plague!"

The plague played a crucial role in the shift from the medieval to the modern world during the mid- to late fourteenth century in Florence, the birthplace of Renaissance thought. There the Black Death, which struck in 1347, killed at least 50 percent (and possibly as much as 80

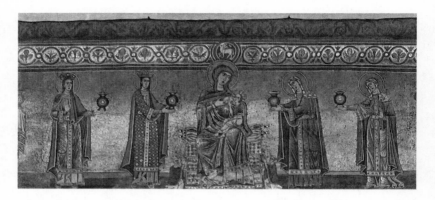

4. A twelfth-century mosaic, depicting Mary breastfeeding the infant Jesus, on the façade of the Basilica di Santa Maria in Trastevere (Rome, Italy). https://commons .wikimedia.org/wiki/File:Exterior_Mosiac_of_Santa_Maria_Trastevere.jpg

percent) of the population. The resulting demographic shift created new spaces for mobility, and people moved to cities like Florence to take advantage of new economic opportunities.

The horrors of the plague shook religious faith, prefiguring the end of chivalric values and the rise of mercantile capitalism. Some people became even more devout, but others pursued a kind of secular humanism, a move reflected in the rise of realism in literature, philosophy, and other fields. For example, *The Decameron* (Boccaccio [1351] 2003) describes Florentine aristocrats telling each other stories as they flee the plague over a ten-day period, but in the introduction Boccaccio, having lived through it, describes the disease in dreadful, real-life detail. In art and philosophy Alberti extols the self as something you cultivate, an idea that departed radically from being born into a station (Tanabe 2016; Alberti [1438] 1751). By 1486 Giovanni Pico della Mirandola had penned his *Oration on the Dignity of Man*, often referred to as the "Manifesto of the Italian Renaissance," which called for veneration of the human mind and potential for achievement.

This shift was significant for art too; rather than a continuation of stylized icons of saints, there is a move toward realistic images. Religious figures become embodied, more humanized, as in Donatello's *David* (1440). The Nursing Madonna is caught up in this transition, which is why we begin to see the Madonna rendered as a humanized mother,

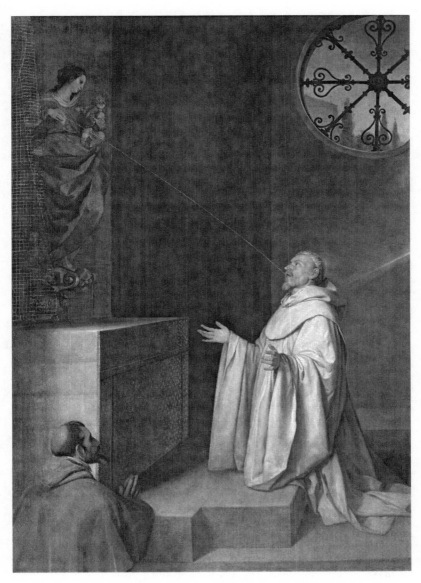

5. Alonso Cano, *The Miraculous Lactation of Saint Bernard*, c. 1650. http://theological anthropology.com/alphabet-of-love/2013/11/7/roman-love-caritas-romana /

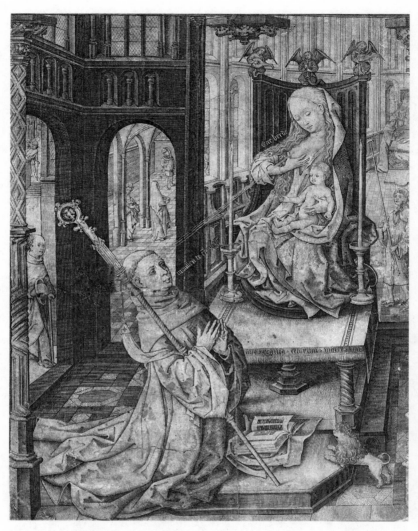

6. Master I.A.M. of Zwoll, *The Lactation of St. Bernard*, 1480–85. The Virgin Mary is shooting milk into the eye of Saint Bernard from her left breast. Bernard himself described in the twelfth century this miraculous healing of an eye affliction.
https://commons.wikimedia.org/wiki/File:StBernardFS.jpg.

a mother nursing her baby. In celebration of ooze, Mary's dripping milk marks her humanness.

In a myth extolling the miracle of lactation Saint Bernard asks the Madonna to show herself as Mother. She obliges, spraying breast milk onto his face, at times across a quite impressive distance.[3] (People continue to squirt breast milk—as a miraculous healing elixir—into babies' eyes or up their noses to ward off infections.)

Following the condemnation of nudity in religious subjects by the Council of Trent (1545–63), Madonna Lactans starts to disappear. In "Disrobing the Virgin: The *Madonna Lactans* in Fifteenth-Century Florentine Art" Megan Holmes (1997) argues that rising naturalism made depicting the breast increasingly problematic, with Madonna Lactans imagery waning from the 1740s on.

The seeping maternal body has yet to be fully redeemed. As Miranda explained it to me, "the appearance of the Lactating Madonna in art is kind of an anomaly because although there was a Dionysian opportunity to celebrate the body, Renaissance artists ultimately privileged the Apollonian, so I see the exploration of the Madonna as a real woman to be a kind of branch cut short. She starts to appear as a real lactating woman, but then she becomes idealized. Airbrushed like contemporary celebrities! Celebrities are not often shown breastfeeding because it transforms them from icon to mama. It makes them real." Apparently celebrities in American society, like late medieval Madonnas, should not be depicted in any of their leaky glory.

The performance of motherhood, care, and healing power through lactation, as well as themes of the sacred, sexuality and the body, the abject, circulation, and commodification that are ringing throughout these historical images emerges again in the 2000s within the context of breast milk sharing.

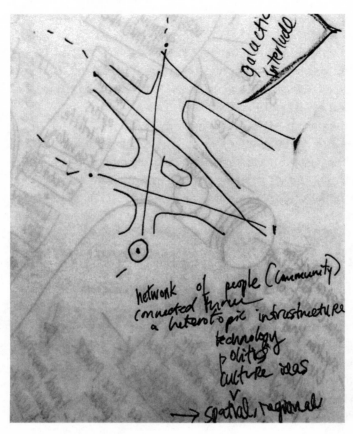

7. Notebook sketch by author.

1   Milk Moves

When I explained to our neighbor that I needed to borrow their cooler because I was taking a road trip to Jacksonville to pick up a stash of frozen breast milk, Allie's reaction was one of wide-eyed surprise and curiosity: "What?! You can do that?" As a mother of three, she had a lot of questions: "How did you find it? How does it work? Do you have to match each other, you know, by race or something? Or age? Is she a friend? Do you pay her?" Since many others asked these same questions, this chapter describes the mechanics of pumping and storage, as well as how the sharing system works.

Milk

Human milk is, from an evolutionary perspective, a biological norm, a time-tested standard of care providing babies with well-documented benefits such as decreased risk of infection and protection against allergies, asthma, arthritis, diabetes, obesity, cardiovascular disease, and various cancers (Mead 2008; Van Esterik 2011). Breast milk also contains a range of immunoprotective components, including secretory Immunoglobulin A (IgA), lactoferrin, lysozyme, bifidus factor, oligosaccharides, milk lipids, and milk leukocytes (Wagner, Anderson, and Pittard 1996).

Mothers' milk is not unique to humans, but the synthesis of milk in mammary glands, which are a kind of modified sweat gland, is the defining characteristic of mammals, so understanding its role during critical periods of development in infancy makes milk an important topic of research (Miller et al. 2013). Almost all mammals deliver milk to the young through a teat, or nipple (the two exceptions are the spiny anteater and the platypus, whose babies lick milk off of their mothers' bodies). Below the teat, milk ducts branch out into alveoli, which siphon protein, sugar, and fat from the blood supply for milk production, with full-scale production starting between forty-eight and ninety-six hours after birth, as prolactin levels rise. It is not, as you might have imagined by watching a baby nurse, sucking alone that releases the milk. Nor does it just seep out once it is produced; secretion requires chemical and often physical stimulation. When a mother's milk "lets down," oxytocin and prolactin generate a milk-ejection reflex during which time the alveoli contract and the milk is squeezed out (the nursing baby also stimulates the mother's body to release the hormones that start the let-down).

All milk is not the same—each mother's milk will reflect the conditions of her body—and it changes over time. Milk can contain alcohol, caffeine, or pharmaceutical products that a mother has ingested. It will contain antibodies manufactured by the mother's body in response to her environment. Milk secreted for a new infant—the golden-colored, high-antibody and high-immunoglobulin colostrum—is different from that produced for an older baby. The constitution of milk even changes during a single feeding: foremilk, milk released at the beginning of the feeding, contains less fat than the hindmilk, secreted later in the feeding. As explained by the La Leche League website, milk-making cells

> produce only one type of milk, but the fat content of the milk that is removed varies according to how long the milk has been collecting in the ducts and how much of the breast is drained. . . . As milk is made, the fat sticks to the sides of the milk-making cells while the watery portion of the milk moves down the ducts toward the nipple, where it mixes with any milk left there from the last feeding. The longer the amount of time between feedings, the more diluted that leftover milk becomes. This "watery" milk has a higher lactose content and less fat than the milk stored in the milk-making cells higher up in the breast. As baby begins nursing, the first thing he receives is this lower-fat foremilk, which quenches his thirst. Baby's nursing triggers the mother's milk ejection reflex, which squeezes milk and the sticking fat cells from the milk-making cells into the ducts. This higher-fat hindmilk mixes with the high-lactose foremilk and baby receives the perfect food, with fat calories for growth and lactose for energy and brain development. (La Leche League 2015)

As the baby nurses, or as the mother pumps, the foremilk slowly changes into hindmilk; there is no discrete point of changeover. Babies need both. And some of our donors labeled pumped milk as "foremilk" or "hindmilk" before freezing it so that the two could be combined at our baby's feeding.

All milk cannot go anywhere, any time. The fact that it spoils, that it has a shelf life (even when frozen solid), that it can be bitter or sweet, that not all babies will take all milk, that making milk requires time and energy, that its constitution changes as the baby develops, and that not everyone can produce it, all contribute to determining to whom milk goes and how. Milk comes in a range of colors (white, blue, yellow, and orange) and textures (viscous or thin). Milk with an excess of lipase (an enzyme in breast milk that helps to break down fat) can smell "off" and taste bitter or soapy (and some babies will not drink it). High-lipase milk is perfectly nutritious but unacceptable to some donees. Others may not accept milk from women taking certain medications. I once rejected milk from a donor who was taking Zoloft even though I learned that doctors identified sertraline as one of the preferred drugs for new mothers because it shows up in breast milk in smaller quantities than other selective serotonin reuptake inhibitors (SSRIS) (Berle and Spigset 2011; Weissman et al. 2004). These qualities influence who gets what milk, how much they can have, and what they do with it.

Looking Around

When I first started searching for studies related to sharing, I discovered a small library of popular trade books, most published since 2005, dealing with everything from work and breastfeeding balance in milk production to the sexual body (Colburn-Smith and Serrette 2007; Tamaro 2005; West and Marasco 2008). I also found a few scholarly texts exploring milk contamination (Boswell-Penc 2006) and constructions of nursing in "appropriate" motherhood (Barston 2012; Wolf 2013). Overtly anthropological work has examined breastfeeding historically (Fildes 1987; Whitaker 2000); as it relates to sexuality and mothering (Mabilia 2005; Zeitlyn and Rowshan 1997); from a biological perspective, especially as compared to formula (Draper 1996; Ebrahim 1980; Ryan 1988); as related to fertility (Jelliffe 1976; Finka et al. 1992); in the context of emerging labor and consumer markets (Gottschang 2007); with regard to kinship (Dettwyler 1998; El Guindi 2011, 2012); vis-à-vis mothering (Barlow 2010; Barlow and Chapin 2010); and in HIV-positive contexts (Kroeker and Beckwith 2011; Van Hollen 2011).

More germane to my project was research on milk purchased online (Geraghty et al. 2013; Keim et al. 2013; Keim et al. 2015; Stevens and Keim 2015; Stuebe, Gribble, and Palmquist 2014) and some excellent anthropological work based on an analysis of sharing as presented in newspapers as risky and irresponsible (Reyes-Foster, Carter, and Rogers 2015) and from surveys and interviews with donors and donees (Carroll 2015b; Palmquist and Doehler 2014, 2016; Reyes-Foster, Carter, and Hinojosa 2015). What I did not find were in-depth ethnographic studies.

There is, however, plenty of work on the related practice of allo-mothering, which is carrying, providing food, or guarding another mother's offspring from predators, particularly among primates such as vervets, squirrel monkeys, and macaques. The practice of women providing milk for other mothers' babies, or allo-nursing (what we would call "wet-nursing" in a human context), has been observed in many mammals, not just humans. Perhaps there is some kind of adaptive advantage at play, but further research is needed to adequately understand the functions, costs, and benefits for both babies and adults. The act of nursing, for example, may confer advantages (such as fostering a mother-baby emotional connection) while receiving milk without nursing (through the help of technology such as bottles) may confer others (e.g., nutritional benefits). But even when we do identify the functions, costs, and benefits of milk sharing in primate populations at large, they may or may not all apply in the same way to humans.

A panel at the 2010 American Anthropology Association (AAA) annual meeting focused on a related question. The panel, entitled "Human Consumption of 'Afterbirth' (Maternal Placentophagy): A Natural and Beneficial Practice?," explored the eating of placenta among humans, which is conspicuously absent from the cross-cultural record but ubiquitous among nearly all other terrestrial mammals (save camels). In the United States, where this practice is on the rise, it is sometimes legitimated by referring to it as an "ancient Chinese custom," which reflects a cultural stereotype of Chinese medicine as bizarre yet effective, rather than being based on anything verifiable. Pierre Leinard (2010) reported in this panel that his research in the Human Relations Area Files turned up no evidence showing human placentophagy as a customary practice in any known contemporary or historic cultures.[4]

Other AAA panelists raised questions about placentophagy's absence (or extreme rarity) in prehistoric and historic populations and contemporary human cultures against a small but visible trend in the United States (Benyshek 2010). In her paper on placentophagy and the U.S. home birth movement, Melissa Cheyney (2010) has argued that "rituals of the early postpartum period at home including placental examination, celebration, disposal and consumption are intentionally constructed by midwives to communicate messages to mothers about the sufficiency of the birthing body, as well as the sacredness or miraculous quality of their home deliveries." Apparently among home-birth proponents the practice has perceived, if not real, benefits that range from replenishing iron and enhancing lactation to beating back the "baby blues." Cheyney even provides pictures of lasagna and other dishes prepared with placental materials.

Some breast milk sharing participants I worked with were also involved in placentophagy: one donor is a regional "go-to" source for drying the placenta and for making placenta art, and another had her placenta encapsulated for future consumption. Interestingly, Sharon Young and Daniel Benyshek (2010) have shown that the hormonal and nutritional content of the human placenta, particularly in dehydrated and encapsulated forms, has not been established.

As with placentophagy, claims about breast milk need further investigation. Because a mother's milk contains antibodies, drinking milk made by many different women could, theoretically, introduce a larger swath of antibodies to the baby. This was an idea I heard repeated by many donors and donees. Even friends who had heard about milk sharing suggested that enhanced antibody diversity was a possible benefit. A review of current research suggests that milk not only serves immunological functions but also contains factors with a variety of biological roles: milk contains hormones, growth factors, enzymes, lactoferrin, lysozyme, oligosaccharides, nucleotides, antioxidants, and other cellular components that protect against infection, exert an immunomodulant effect, and support beneficial intestinal bacterial flora (Giuliani et al. 2014).

Notable constituents of mature human milk include:

WATER

FAT

- Myristic acid
- Palmitic acid
- Linoleic acid
- Alpha-linolenic acid
- Arachidonic acid
- Docosahexaenoic acid

PROTEIN

- Whey protein
- Casein protein

HORMONES

- Leptin
- Ghrelin
- Adiponectin
- Insulin
- Insulinlike growth factor-1 (IGF-1)
- Insulinlike growth factor-2 (IGF-2)
- Cortisol

IMMUNE FACTORS

- Secretory IgA (sIgA)
- Lactoferrin
- Lysozyme
- Transforming growth factor beta (TGFβ)
- Interleukin 1 (IL-1)
- Interleukin 6 (IL-6)
- Interleukin 10 (IL-10)
- Tumor necrosis factor alpha (TNF-α)

CARBOHYDRATES

- Lactose
- Oligosaccharides

ASH

- Vitamin A
- Vitamin D

Calcium
Phosphorus
Iron
Zinc
Copper (Miller et al. 2013, 2)

Policy

Today powerful institutions promote breastfeeding or suggest that women offer a combination of breastfeeding and feeding babies mothers' milk. Citing documented long-term and short-term neurodevelopmental advantages, the American Academy of Pediatrics (AAP) began in 2005 to advance breastfeeding and human milk as normative standards for infant feeding and nutrition and recommended exclusive breastfeeding for six months, followed by continued breastfeeding as complementary foods are introduced, with the continuation of breastfeeding for one year or longer as mutually desired by mother and infant. The AAP recognizes contraindications for breastfeeding, such as when the mother has an active, untreated case of tuberculosis or is actively using drugs such as phencyclidine (commonly known as PCP), cannabis, or cocaine.

A 2011 AAP report showed that almost 75 percent of all American women initiate breastfeeding, but this figure obscures some significant demographic information. For example, the rate for breastfeeding in Hispanic populations is about 80 percent, while only about 58 percent of African American mothers initiate breastfeeding. Among mothers participating in the federal Women, Infants, and Children supplemental nutrition program, initiating breastfeeding rates were 67.5 percent overall, but for those with a higher income the rate was 84.6 percent. For low-income non-Hispanic African American mothers the rate was only 37 percent. Older mothers were more likely to breastfeed. The lowest rates of initiation were among non-Hispanic African American mothers younger than twenty, for whom the breastfeeding initiation rate was only 30 percent. The highest rates for exclusive breastfeeding are among urban, white, well-educated women with higher incomes.[5]

If we were to look six months out from the initiation point, the "any breastfeeding" rate in 2011 was 43 percent (with Hispanic or Latinas at 46 percent and non-Hispanic African Americans at 27 percent). Only 13 percent of the mothers met the recommendation to breastfeed exclusively for six months. So as a national population Americans are a long way from the AAP goal, significant internal demographic differences notwithstanding. But why? For one thing, disparities in breastfeeding rates are associated with variations in hospital routines, including when and how formula is presented to new mothers. Other factors implicated in disparities include the media, which often cite difficulties with breastfeeding rather than positive stories, different policies on work and parental leave, social and cultural norms, and advice from family and friends (U.S. Surgeon General 2011). I suspect that there is much more to it, and while this is not a study of breastfeeding per se, demographic differences identified by these reports were strongly reflected in my milk-sharing community, which comprises largely white, educated, and middle-class women who are well aware of the AAP policy.

The policy echoes *Breastfeeding and Maternal and Infant Health Outcomes in Developed Countries*, a report prepared by the Evidence-Based Practice Centers of the Agency for Healthcare Research and Quality of the U.S. Department of Health and Human Services (Ip et al. 2007). The AAP identifies this report as the most comprehensive analysis of scientific literature comparing breastfeeding to formula. It shows that the risk of hospitalization for lower respiratory tract infections is reduced by 72 percent in the first year for infants breastfed exclusively for more than four months and that *any* breastfeeding is associated with a 64 percent reduction of nonspecific gastrointestinal tract infections (an effect that lasts for two months after cessation of breastfeeding). Exclusive breastfeeding for three to four months helps reduce the incidence of clinical asthma, atopic dermatitis, and eczema by 27 percent in low-risk populations and up to 42 percent in infants with a family history of these conditions. Finally, there is a reduction of 52 percent in the risk of developing celiac disease in infants breastfed at the time of gluten exposure, a 31 percent reduction in the risk of childhood inflammatory bowel disease, significantly lower rates of obesity, up to a 30 percent reduction in the incidence of type 1 diabetes mellitus in infants exclusively breastfed for at least three months, and a reduction in leukemia that is correlated with the duration of breastfeeding (Eidelman and Schanler 2012).

The case for providing human milk to preterm infants is extremely compelling, according to this study, with regard to preventing necrotizing enterocolitis and promoting growth and neurodevelopment. Breastfeeding also affects maternal health: for example, breastfeeding is associated with decreased postpartum blood loss and more rapid involution of the uterus, while breastfeeding (cumulatively) for twelve to twenty-three months is associated with significant reduction in rates of hypertension, hyperlipidemia, cardiovascular disease, and diabetes. Breastfeeding is also thought to reduce the risk of both breast and ovarian cancers.

In light of this research current AAP policy reaffirms the group's 2005 call to breastfeed and states that since breastfeeding and the use of human milk confer unique nutritional and non-nutritional benefits to both infant and mother and optimize infant, child, and adult health as well as child growth and development, infant feeding should not be considered a lifestyle choice but rather a basic health issue. The group also indicates that the pediatrician's role in advocating and supporting proper breastfeeding practices is essential and vital for the achievement of the preferred public health goal of exclusive breastfeeding for six months and beyond (Eidelman and Schanler 2012, e837). These recommendations are shared by the U.S. Department of Health and Human Services, the U.S. Surgeon General, the Centers for Disease Control (CDC), the World Health Organization (WHO), and the Institute of Medicine, and they underpin globally distributed hospital protocol such as the WHO/UNICEF's "Ten Steps to Successful Breastfeeding," which prioritizes breastfeeding, or at least breast milk, over formula (World Health Organization 2009).

Structural regulations and hospital practices can support breastfeeding. For example, public hospitals run by the New York City Health and Hospitals Corporation banned formula bags and promotional materials in 2007, and twelve private New York City hospitals made the same move when they signed on to the city's Latch On initiative; thirty of the nation's forty-five top-ranked hospitals have stopped distributing formula samples and formula company–sponsored discharge bags.[6]

Civic groups also promote breastfeeding. La Leche League International, founded in the United States in 1956, is the most powerful nongovernmental organization actively influencing attitudes and practices

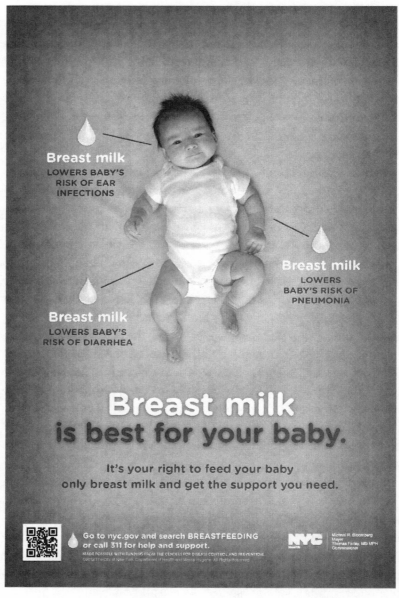

8. The New York City Health Department's "Breast milk is best for your baby" poster campaign describes the benefits of breast milk: reducing the risk of ear infections, diarrhea, and pneumonia. Courtesy of the New York City Department of Health and Mental Hygiene.

related to breast milk. Echoing AAP policy, the stated mission of LLL is to help mothers worldwide to breastfeed through mother-to-mother support, encouragement, information, and education and to promote a better understanding of breastfeeding as an important element in the healthy development of the baby and mother. La Leche League meetings are held in every state, are free and open to everyone, and provide support and training to new (and experienced) moms. And while some donees I talked with criticized LLL for being "too militant," others credited the support gained by attending LLL meetings as part of the reason they were able to pump successfully. So great was their gratitude, some planned to become involved in LLL leadership. This makes sense insofar as LLL has prioritized grassroots-level work aimed at helping individual mothers to breastfeed.

So while there is an overwhelming public call to support feeding infants with breast milk, none of these organizations supports what they call peer-to-peer or informal breast milk sharing, citing health risks. In reality the study of both informally shared milk and the impact of receiving breast milk from the breast as opposed to receiving it by the bottle remains scant.

Meanwhile investment in research on breast milk is intensifying, in part to discover more about the economic ramifications of use in terms of infant care but also in terms of the commercial possibilities. For example, because of the costs associated with necrotizing enterocolitis (NEC), a dangerous condition in which intestinal tissue begins to die, a lot of research focuses on infants in neonatal intensive care units who until recently were fed formula. Breast milk seems to stave off NEC as compared to formula, so providing pasteurized human milk to NICU babies is on the rise (Carroll 2012). The benefits of breast milk over formula for very low birth weight and other high-risk infants are also now considered "well established"; infants fed breast milk are said to display improved feeding tolerance and develop fewer severe infections and fewer episodes of NEC and bronchopulmonary dysplasia. They have improved cardiovascular health and fewer pathogenic organisms, experience shorter hospital stays with reduced rates of hospital readmission, and show improved neurodevelopmental outcomes (Panczuk et al. 2014; Giuliani et al. 2014).

This is all wonderful from the point of view of parents, but there is also a bottom line: it is less expensive to care for healthier infants. The clear clinical evidence for improved outcomes for preterm infants provided with milk means that demand for insurance or state-funded banked milk is increasing since not all NICU mothers can provide milk to their new babies. At present there is far more demand than supply, and milk banks are working to increase their inventories.

Labor and Science

It is important not to underestimate role of modernity (and postmodernity) in the rise and fall of breastfeeding, especially with regard to technology and the construction of women as gendered subjects, as parents, and as laborers. In the realm of milk, modernity brought us milk stations, formula, milk banks, polluted milk, and now breast milk sharing.

From the late nineteenth century until the 1920s the U.S. labor force contained relatively few married women; although there were some professionals, women were largely doing piecework in manufacturing or working in the service industry as domestics and laundresses, and they often left the workforce when they married (Goldin 2006). Claudia Goldin points out that many jobs available to women were dirty, repetitive, or dangerous and that there was a substantial social stigma to working outside the home.

By the late 1920s laws in most municipalities ensured that cow's milk was processed in sanitary conditions. As pasteurized milk was hailed as safe for young and old, mothers gave their babies cow's milk (despite pleas from health officials to breastfeed). The introduction of milk substitutes in the 1920s and 1930s exerted additional pressure against breastfeeding, and many women, both those who worked and those who stayed home, started to view it as a matter of lifestyle. Embracing technology, women also began giving birth in hospitals instead of at home (Mead 2008).

The 1950s witnessed a celebration of the rise of science. Atomic-era ideology promised that new forms of knowledge would liberate society, and even reproduction and parenting were brought under the purview of experts in a culture of "scientific motherhood" (Avishai 2011, 24). Many mothers (as now) were diagnosed with "insufficient milk syndrome" and told by pediatricians to give their babies formula, touted as not only modern, convenient, and nutritionally equivalent but also as superior (Avishai 2011, 24). Breastfeeding reached an all-time low in 1956 of about 20 percent.[7]

Perhaps it is not that surprising that from the 1930s to the 1970s, during the rise of the chemical age and when the demand for clerical and other office work grew (some of which was wartime or part-time work), milk substitutes became increasingly popular. Early in this period women were still leaving the workforce when they married (and had children), "in part because of the institution of marriage bans, regulations that forced single women to leave employment upon marriage and barred the hiring of married women" in school districts and clerical fields, but as these bans were eliminated (after the 1940s), the workforce swelled (Goldin 2006, 5). Concomitantly stigmas about women (even those who were married with children) working outside the home began to fade. Scholars have pointed out that the rise in "insufficient milk syndrome" was actually the direct result of "expert" practices such as postparturition infant-mother separation and breastfeeding schedules that interfered with lactation (Apple 1987). During the same time period the seeds for a feminist critique of science were being sown: in 1963 LLL published *The Womanly Art of Breastfeeding*, which contained a reappraisal of formula.

By the 1970s not only were medical and pharmaceutical practitioners revisiting the value of breast milk but breastfeeding had begun, slowly, to regain acceptance. During this era my sister and I were both fed formula, a choice my mother made by following social customs, but, reflecting a shift in attitudes, my brother, born five years later, was breastfed.

Women's participation in the labor force continued to grow, partly because women expected to have a career that would shape their identity (rather than seeking intermittent or short-lived work), began to marry later, and were more likely to consider divorce, all of which changed how young women planned for a secure future (Goldin 2006). But additional pharmaceutical, technological, and legal issues were also at play.

One such issue was the rollout of the oral contraceptive; "the Pill" gave women more control over their reproductive life. Many chose to work first and then marry and have children later. Pump technology enabled women with children, even very young children, to work and continue to breastfeed. By the 1980s new mothers could hire a lactation consultant: not only had knowledge about breastfeeding been lost in previous generations, but instruction in breastfeeding was becoming professionalized, even monetized. An ever-expanding array of nipple creams, nursing bras, pads, pillows, pumps, and advice books was offered to those with money to spare.

Still, even in 2001 a study by Joan Meek in *Pediatric Clinics of North America* concluded that only about 10 percent of working mothers provided any breast milk to their six-month-old infants, compared to about 30 percent of stay-at-home mothers who did so, a difference of about 20 percent that she found to be consistent across ethnic, educational, and age groups. With the passage of the 2010 Patient Protection and Affordable Care Act (PPACA) these figures are now higher, but even with the mandate for lactation facilities in the workplace in place only a little more than a quarter of full-time and a third of part-time working mothers still breastfeed at six months.

So while there has been a widening acceptance of breastfeeding since the 1990s, problems remain. Pam Carter's (1995) *Feminism, Breasts and Breast-Feeding* challenges the "breast milk is best" narrative, arguing that it functions to critique and police poor, African American, and less-educated mothers' bodies and that it fails to consider the varied meanings and experiences of breastfeeding among different populations. Linda Blum's (1999) *At the Breast* delivers a searing critique of LLL and the failure of proponents of exclusive breastfeeding to deal with class issues related to who can choose to breastfeed.

Clearly the political economy of childcare has to be considered: short and/or poorly paid maternity leave for most women (and almost non-existent paternity leave) combined with little support for lactating women in the workplace makes it hard for most women to breastfeed for the recommended time period. Poor, less-educated, and minority women tend to have difficulty complying with the AAP regimen and may resist it as an imposition of white, middle-class mothering standards (Avishai 2011). Even if you can pay for the services of a lactation consultant and have sufficient privacy and support for breastfeeding and pumping, deciding between formula and breast milk is not simple.

But what about nonlactating moms who choose breast milk? Despite the vehement claim that "breast milk is best," powerful institutions are opposed to the informal milk sharing this book explores.[8] What's a parent to do?

Wet-Nursing

I do not mind sharing my own naïveté: when our doula, Issa, suggested donated milk for our baby, my own response was, "You can really do that?" I knew about allo-mothering, but for some reason I thought milk was like blood: it had to be matched to the baby. Our doula does not suffer fools gladly, but she endured me: "My dear, have you ever heard of a wet nurse? Me and my sistas, we always nursed each other's kids." And really, this is not so different. "Okay," I said, curious and eager to explore the idea. "So how does that work"? I was pretty sure that I would not be looking for a wet nurse since, as far as I knew, the profession had all but disappeared.

When people were unable or unwilling to breastfeed, families, at least as far back as 2000 BCE, could hire a wet nurse.[9] As opposed to cross-feeding (the informal sharing of breastfeeding between equals that is usually unpaid and sometimes reciprocal, as Issa had described), wet-nursing was typically done by an employer's social inferior, was never reciprocal (the hiring mother did not wet-nurse the nurse's children), and was normally done in exchange for payment (Thorley 2008).

During the eighteenth and nineteenth centuries wet nurses were common in England and Europe, especially among the French aristocracy. From the end of the eighteenth century through the nineteenth century, with the onset of the Industrial Revolution and urban migration, the practice of wet-nursing shifted away from wealthy families to laboring, lower-income families. This shift occurred when an increased cost of living combined with low wages forced many women to seek employment, making it virtually impossible for them to breastfeed their children, who were consequently farmed out to destitute peasants (Osborn 1979). Eighteenth-century medical critiques such as William Buchan's *Domestic Medicine* (1769) advanced a distrust of wet nurses and their use of tinctures such as the opiate-based Godfrey's Cordial to quiet crying infants.[10] This was happening at the same time that bottle technology was improving, safer cow's milk was more readily available,

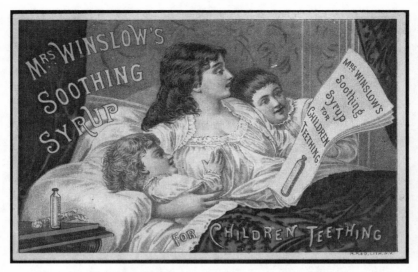

9. Similar to Godfrey's Cordial, made with coriander, anise, treacle, and opium, Mrs. Winslow's Soothing Syrup contained morphine. http://ark
.digitalcommonwealth.org/ark:/50959/8k71nj083.

and the acceptability and quality of formula were on the rise (Stevens, Patrick, and Pickler 2009). By 1900 wet-nursing as an organized profession was on its way out (Wickes 1953).

In "Fresh Milk" Fiona Giles (2003) writes that in the United States wet-nursing was common into the 1940s, with directories set up in Boston, New York, and Philadelphia by doctors who promoted regulated wet-nursing over what they saw as the use of inferior cow's milk–based alternatives. But as medical opinion turned away from wet-nursing toward formula, doctors exploited the Victorian notion that "breast-feeding was unrefined, even beastly" (Giles 2003, 22). And technology had come a long way in terms of feeding devices and substitute milks.[11]

Milk Stations

Women in all echelons of American and European society moved away from the wet nurse and began to supplement their own supply with cow's milk. Some avoided breastfeeding altogether, and, among those who did breastfeed, many weaned babies before three months of age (Mead 2008). "Hand-feeding" with unhygienically processed cow's milk

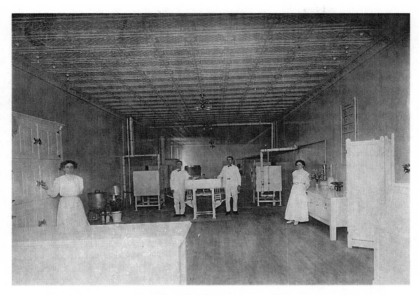

10. Nathan Straus's pasteurized milk laboratory, Washington DC. Library of Congress, Prints and Photographs Division, LC-DIG-ggbain-08157. http://www.loc.gov/pictures/item/ggb2004008157/.

led to high infant mortality rates in urban centers like New York (and elsewhere), especially among poor populations in which women returned to work shortly after giving birth. A fascinating historical intervention in infant feeding came in the form of milk stations.

In their descriptively titled book *Infant Mortality and Milk Stations: Special Report Dealing with the Problem of Reducing Infant Mortality, Work carried on in Ten Largest Cities in the United States together With Details of a Demonstration Held by Private and Public Agencies in New York City During 1911 To Determine the Value of Milk Station Work As A Practical Means of Reducing Infant Mortality*, Philip Van Ingen and Paul Taylor (1912, 22) describe how the Good Samaritan Dispensary, founded in 1891, dispensed milk "modified to a set formula, suited to a definite age, and pasteurized" in the summer when infant mortality was highest. By 1898 the dispensary was operating year round.

Nathan Straus, cofounder of Macy's, decided to take personal action against the "white peril": raw, contaminated milk that was believed to be a factor in child deaths (two of Straus's own children had died at a young age). Urban people of means could keep a cow in a private stable, but the middle class and the poor had to buy milk brought in from rural farms. It was often of poor quality and contaminated with bacterial growth. Believing that Louis Pasteur's new technique of heating milk to kill bacteria was the answer, Straus built his own pasteurization plant on East Third Street in 1893. He eventually opened eighteen stations where any mother could obtain "a safe, well prepared milk, the formulae being provided by the best medical authorities in the city" (Van Ingen and Taylor 1912, 28). Infant mortality rates decreased in milk station areas. Raw milk sales were banned, and city agencies began managing supply to reduce infant mortality among the poorest populations. By 1918 all states had laws requiring that milk for sale be pasteurized. This policy had a profound impact on infant mortality.

Milk banks are similar to milk stations in that they carry low-priced or free pasteurized human milk. The first English milk bank was established in 1935, when a nurse at Queen Charlotte's Hospital organized milk to be collected for a set of quadruplets born there; the scheme was so successful that a formal milk bank was established four years later; by the early twenty-first century there were more than thirteen milk banks operating in England (Giles 2003).

In the United States the first milk bank opened in 1910 at the Boston Floating Hospital. By 1929 banks had been established in at least twenty American cities (Golden 1996). Women sold milk to these banks (up through the 1950s), earning between twenty-five and one hundred dollars per month. As formula feeding became more popular, banks bought less milk, and middle-class women started to donate it. By the 1980s the supply consisted entirely of donations, marking a turn toward the construction of milk as a precious and sacred gift that, like organ or blood donation, should not be treated as a commodity.

During the 1980s many banks closed in response to rising concerns about disease transmission, especially with regard to HIV (Panczuk et al. 2014). As testing improved and powerful organizations touted the value of breast milk, banks began operating again, this time under the Human Milk Banking Association of North America (HMBANA) umbrella. Organized in 1985, HMBANA had as its mission to promote the health of babies and mothers by providing safe pasteurized donor milk and supporting breastfeeding. HMBANA regulates the quality and distribution of donated milk with mandatory guidelines and inspections of member milk banks.

Currently at least twenty-four banks distribute milk in the United States and Canada, and there are more in various stages of development.[12] These banks seek donations from lactating moms who are breastfeeding or from mothers whose babies have died. They do not generally accept milk from those who have induced lactation (as some milk sellers are now doing).

Donors are screened for HIV, human T-cell lymphotropic virus (HTLV), syphilis, and hepatitis B and C. Donated milk undergoes complex processing.[13] Treated milk is tested for contamination; once it passes inspection, it is mixed with other milks, frozen, and dispensed. Because advances in medical technology help more babies than ever to survive low birth weight and/or extremely premature births, the demand for milk is substantial; banks are scrambling to keep up.

According to the HMBANA website, the association's milk dispensation rose from 409,077 ounces in 2000 to more than 2 million ounces in 2011. These banks, which are nonprofit organizations, absorb the costs of recruiting, shipping, testing, and processing donor milk and then sending it out. Once processed, HMBANA milk costs somewhere between four and ten dollars per ounce (compared to formula, which costs as little as pennies per ounce).

WakeMed, a bank located in North Carolina, sells milk for $5 per ounce, but it is only available with a prescription and health insurers may or may not cover the cost. The South Carolina Milk Bank opened in April 2015 and sells milk for $4 an ounce, but it distributes only to hospitals in South Carolina. When I asked my insurance agent about buying milk from an HMBANA bank, the eventual answer was a resounding "no." I cannot say I was too surprised: a baby might take between twenty-five to thirty-five ounces of milk per day, which could cost more than $1,000 a week. Two donees I interviewed had also approached banks but like me were unable to acquire banked milk for their otherwise healthy children.

HMBANA takes a position similar to that of LLL: despite good intentions, shared milk is unsafe, and thus it is better to give it to a bank, where it can be tested it for safety (Brooks 2012). Could it be that peer-to-peer sharing is viewed as a threat to the already insufficient supply going to milk banks? Distribution protocols send banked milk almost exclusively to sick or severely underweight preemies in NICU units, while those receiving milk through informal shares are children who do not qualify for it. But maybe sharing helps rather than harms milk bank supplies: Akre, Gribble, and Minchin (2011) argue that the expanding network of breast milk sharing might benefit milk banking by increasing awareness of the significance and availability of breast milk, persuading more qualifying mothers to donate, and thereby actually increasing banked supplies. I would add that another challenge to banks' supply is the rise in for-profit companies such as Prolacta that pay donors for their milk (but then sell it for a substantial profit). On the other hand, several donors I talked with explained they had worked with or attempted to work with nonprofit HMBANA banks but would never do so for a for-profit company. In my sharing community the notion of selling milk, especially to a for-profit corporation, was explicitly frowned upon. Other values were tacit, but it took time to figure out what those values were.

Sharing

There are two ways to locate donor milk. One is by word of mouth, which is how our doula connected us with Haylee, one of our first donors. Haylee introduced us to women in her circle, but she also showed us the second way to acquire milk: the Internet. There are now at least three established websites—Facebook, MilkShare, and Only the Breast—that connect parents who have extra milk with those who need it (and, as will become obvious, the importance of digital technology to this practice cannot be understated).

Parents can also use local Facebook parenting pages to donate or ask for milk. Some local pages are private, and membership maybe be limited or curated by an administrator, so joining requires making a special request: for example, Milky Mommas, a support group for moms near Savannah, is only for women.

My husband and I studied the online message boards to understand how it was done. Acquiring milk was a team effort that required posting on multiple sites, reading offers, asking for medical records, doing research, buying milk bags, calling donors, locating dry ice, driving all over the place to pick up milk, and so forth. It was a labor of love, but it consumed lots of time and energy. I am pretty sure I could not have done it alone, and I want to emphasize that not everyone has a partner, the time, or the means to procure milk via sharing.

The Facebook page Haylee first showed us was called Eats on Feets at the time but shortly thereafter changed its name to Human Milk for Human Babies (HM4HB). As the Facebook page explains it, this global network exists "to promote the nourishment of babies and children around the world with human milk. We are dedicated to fostering community between local families who have chosen to share breastmilk."[14] Individual states have one or more HM4HB Facebook pages, depending on the size of the group in the state and whether there are closed pages in addition to public ones. Georgia has two: one is an open, public page, and one is a closed group (people must ask to join and must be approved by a moderator; only people in the group can see postings on that page). We also consulted HM4HB Facebook pages for North Carolina, South Carolina, and Florida. When we went out of town, we easily used pages in Arizona and California to find donors. There are also pages for Canada, Australia, New Zealand, Europe, the UK, and the Virgin Islands, as well as Bali, Croatia, Puerto Rico, Japan, and more.

Both donors' and donees' posts on HM4HB are reviewed by a site administrator. Posts, offering milk read like this:

LINDSAY: I have around 250 ounces to donate in Macon. I'm on a non-restricted diet and no medications. Some has [sic] colostrum. The oldest bag is from the end of January or beginning of February.

—

TAMELA: I've been breastfeeding for two years now with my boys and I make too much for my baby. I'm really interested in sharing—I didn't know that there were woman [sic] out there who wanted it! I have a hand pump. But nothing to store the milk in. I live in Augusta. If you want some, I make plenty! Let me know, we can arrange something! Thanks!

—

SHAWN: I have a small amount of breastmilk (34 ounces) to donate. It was pumped in January 2015, when my daughter was one– three weeks old. Preemie or newborn beneficiary preferred, but happy to help anyone I can! I ate dairy at the time. No medications. Based in Athens, GA.

As you can see, women provide different kinds of information, and although posts are pithy, common elements include how much milk is available, how old it is, how old the mother's own children are, what kinds of medications she takes, information about her diet, whether she needs supplies, where she is located, and so forth.

Postings from donees are also to the point, typically indicating what they need, along with information about why they need it, sometimes disclosing health of the mother and/or child. At times parents note allergies or specify that milk should not contain caffeine, alcohol, nicotine, or drugs. Requests read like this:

JULIANN: Hi all. I am looking for a donor in or near the Macon area. My 4 month old daughter has been EBF [exclusively breastfed] since birth and for some reason I have had an issue with pumping enough to build up any kind of stash. I have enough for a couple of days, but with me returning to work on Monday I'm starting to stress out. I tried formula once and he [*sic*] threw it right back up. If anyone can help I'd be super appreciative!

—

RAQUELLE: I am desperately seeking a milk donor in or near the Marietta area. My 3-month-old son has yet to have breastmilk and I want badly to provide it for him. Please PM me if you are willing to donate, it would be GREATLY appreciated!

—

LEIGH: I have a health condition that prevents me from safely nursing. I produce milk but it is unsafe for me to nurse. I have yet to receive any offers, and have reached out with no luck yet.

Please, I am desperate. Any donations would be a blessing. He is the only one of my three children that has not had breastmilk and it saddens me to not provide this for him.

Posts are not meant to be exhaustive; they only disclose enough information to make an initial impression on potential partners. Details are exchanged in private emails and phone calls.

A second website, MilkShare, describes itself as "an informational resource to help you learn about milk donation and to connect families who can help each other."[15] In addition to message boards MilkShare contains detailed information about building up a milk supply, hygiene techniques, freezing and storage, shipping, and even home pasteurization. The site emphasizes that, when possible, mothers should learn to make their own milk before using donor milk, since donors must work hard to provide milk for those with "true needs" due to surgery, adoption, surrogacy, and so forth.

This implied hierarchy of neediness plays out in posts on both Milk-Share and HM4HB. In the HM4MB posts above you can see Leigh stating, for example, that to demonstrate "true need" she has mentioned a medical condition preventing her from safely nursing.

Sometimes we reached out to donors who seemed like a good match for us, while at other times donors contacted us after seeing our post. The initial contact email often looked similar to this one we received from Olivia:

I have some frozen milk I need to donate so I was wondering if you could use mine. I have frozen bags dating between Sept. 2012 and Jan 2013. My son was born in July 2012. I have no dietary restrictions, don't smoke or do drugs, and have only been taking a multi-vitamin. In October I was on antibiotics but dumped all the milk associated with that week. I'm guessing I have 150 oz. available. Please let me know if this would work for you. I'm located in Guyton at xxx-xxxx. I could also bring it to work (but you'd need to pick up in the morning since there's no freezer there).

Olivia describes when the milk was pumped, the age of her baby, her diet and drug status, vitamin intake, how much frozen—not fresh—milk she has available, and where she is located, clearly the hallmark of someone who has experience doing this. In subsequent communications Olivia and I traded phone numbers, full names, and addresses. Donees may ask for copies of medical records, for information about how the milk was pumped and stored, or whether she would like to be a one-time or regular donor.

Acknowledging that every family is unique and must make its own decisions about making a "milky match," MilkShare recommends that donors be screened for a variety of health concerns, including HIV, hepatitis, syphilis, and human T-cell lymphotropic viruses (milk banks also screen for these viruses) and states that blood work should be reasonably current. The site further recommends that milk from donors who do not meet all blood-screening criteria should be rejected. Furthermore it advises that milk from mothers on medications that can pass through breast milk, who are unwilling to have their blood tested, who cannot or will not provide a complete health history, or who have an "unhealthy" lifestyle should also be rejected.

Donees make their own decisions about which guidelines to follow on a case-by-case basis. Once donors and donees are connected, they work together to see if they are a good fit. We usually requested screening for HIV, hepatitis, syphilis, and HTLV, but not everyone was willing or able to provide this. Piper, a potential donor, wrote to us in an email that in examining her records

> I could only find basic blood tests verifying glucose, hematocrit, blood type, etc. Nothing covered the medical screens you are looking for. Honestly, since I don't know you, I'm not comfortable having my physician fax your [sic] my personal records. As far as, I know I do not have any of the viruses listed. I'm sure it would have been mentioned to me as I've had two children. Other than your typical pet and pollen allergies and a bad back from carrying the baby, I've never had any major medical issues. The only thing in my recent history is a minor case of shingles since I had chicken pox as a kid. The only other thing about my frozen milk is that it can have a slight soapy taste compared to fresh. If you're still interested in the milk, I'm happy to discuss by phone. Please call me up until 11pm at xxx-xxxx.

We did not move forward unless we found an agreeable solution to questions about things like HIV status. In this case Piper ended up bringing to the drop-off a copy of medical records stating that she was HIV negative.

Donors often wanted to know more about our baby and about us: Was it a boy or a girl? Was the baby healthy, or did he have allergies? Was he a good eater and sleeper? How about me, did I work? Why did I adopt? Did I try to induce lactation? I felt like a lot of the time women just wanted to get a sense of where the milk was going, but a few stated outright that they preferred to donate to a baby who was "truly in need," which meant to a family that *could not* breastfeed. We usually stated in our posts that we had an adopted child, and a few donors explained that they had looked for an adopted recipient because they were themselves adopted or had adopted children in their family.

I met other families and even some doulas who used MilkShare's screening forms. On the other hand, some simply went by personal impressions or asked few or sometimes no questions about a donor's lifestyle or health. For example, when Naomi was not able to produce enough milk for her first baby, she gave him formula, but he did not digest it well. So for her second child, Ryan, she used donor milk instead of formula, but she did not use the MilkShare donor agreement. She used an ad hoc approach to learning about her donors, and sometimes she allowed her doula to do the screening for her. Naomi explained,

> Ryan did horrible with it [formula]. He had really bad constipation, and it was hours of screaming every day, and he was sleeping poorly. We found out when he was thirteen months old that he was milk protein intolerant, and the formula was causing him a lot of issues. So when I had low supply with our second, we didn't want to go through all of that again, and felt that donor milk might not cause some of the problems we went through the first time. . . . A few donors I talked to personally, and I asked diet and/or medical questions, but so many were anonymous [coming through my doula] that I didn't know some of that information.

The HM4HB Facebook page is free (once you have Internet access), but recipients in MilkShare pay a one-time joining fee of twenty dollars by PayPal (which admittedly may exclude some people). Neither HM4HB nor MilkShare supports selling breast milk, unlike a third site called Only the Breast (OTB).[16] There, postings called "classifieds" state whether people want to buy, sell, or donate. OTB posts usually list milk for sale, mostly priced between one and three dollars an ounce. But OTB milk is still inexpensive compared to HMBANA prices, and theoretically anyone can purchase it. You can see how an Only the Breast arrangement may be doable for a short-term, supplemental, or emergency situation; most families would not be able to pay what would still amount to many thousands of dollars for milk.

Classifieds on OTB mimic those found on HM4HB and MilkShare, although there are also ads by adult fetishists or other "off-label" requests for milk, such as colostrum for body building or allergy relief. Whether or not and to whom breast milk *should* be sold is hotly debated among many sharing enthusiasts.

Only the Breast is different from both MilkShare and HM4HB in other ways. For example, OTB "requires" milk sold on the site to be home pasteurized (which seems to me to be a very difficult process to follow with any degree of precision).[17]

Besides promoting "home pasteurization" OTB cofounder Glenn Snow is developing the International Milk Bank in Sparks, Nevada, to supply breast milk to hospitals in the United States and overseas, and he promises both "sustainable economic success and enduring shareholder value," which means profits for investors around the globe.[18] In a recent *New York Times* article on the rising commodification of human milk, Snow stated, "It's a fascinating industry, and it's brand-new" (quoted in Pollack 2015).

Donors on all three sites usually offer milk that has already been pumped with a hand or electric pump. Interestingly, and despite the fact that the market for these pumps will reach well over five million units in 2015, these unwieldy, expensive machines have not undergone a major redesign in almost sixty years (Robb 2014). Sometimes donors seek a family that can purchase, rent, or share the cost of a hospital-grade pump in exchange for providing milk over a long period.

Once pumped, milk is frozen in specially designed bags or bottles. The milk can be kept in a regular freezer or deep freezer until it is thawed for use. Most women I met used a six- to twelve-month rule for keeping milk in deep freeze, keeping in mind that, as with cow's milk, as long as it smells and tastes good, it is fine. When in doubt, throw it out.

There are debates about how long milk should be frozen and what impact long- or even short-term freezing has on milk. Hanna et al. (2004) show that antioxidant activity in refrigerated milk is decreased and that freezing results in even greater decreases, with longer storage times being associated with lower antioxidant activity: frozen storage for seven days results in lower antioxidant activity than cold storage for two days. But what, if any, is the practical significance of this loss? The authors point out that even after a week of freezing, human milk still has 25 percent more antioxidant activity than formula. And according to Dermer's (2004) response to this study, despite the loss of antioxidant activity, frozen milk, even when submitted to extremely rigorous freezing routines such as those practiced by milk banks, appears to confer a health advantage to babies when compared to formula.

Expressed milk, fresh or frozen, changes hands in two ways: either during a face-to-face meeting or by post. You cannot transport milk over long distances or mail it without a serious coolant, and, if shipped, it needs to be specially packed and sent rapidly, which can be expensive. In a local exchange the donor and donee meet somewhere—at home or a public place (which may be a kid-friendly park or an innocuous parking lot)—and transfer the milk from one cooler to another.

I met many donors at their own home, bringing my children along. Sometimes the donors came to me, occasionally with their husbands. My husband often drove to meet donors (especially if they lived several hours away, and at least once he recounted a pleasant but slightly awkward meeting with another husband, since, "after all, I was there to pick up something that came out of his wife's breast"). Sometimes a doula or a friend might pick up a stash on their way somewhere else. Naomi reflected,

> I am not sure exactly how many donors we had. I got some of my initial donor milk from my doula, and I don't know how many donors were in there, and a friend and I shared some of the milk that we got. [There were] at least a dozen donors, but it easily could be twice that or more. . . . I became Facebook friends with a woman who transported milk for me. She was a friend of my doula, and transported

milk from six hours away for us. That was our first, and biggest dona-tion. Most of our donors lived three to six hours away. The majority of our milk came in those little two-ounce plastic snappies, so I gave a couple of our donors some of those. Well, I should clarify, "some" was probably a few hundred divided between donors.

I also met women at gas stations, grocery stores, and fast-food restau-rants. These were usually easy-to-identify spots near a major road or highway. (A grocery franchise called Publix usually sells dry ice in Geor-gia, so it was always a convenient meeting point.) Public meet-ups were usually shorter and less intimate than home visits since most people are not too keen on lingering in a hot parking lot with a baby for longer than necessary. Like Naomi, we drove as much as six hours to pick up a large donation, while most out-of-town trips were between two and three hours. Other donees also calculated value in relation to time, driving longer for large or regular donations and not bothering with very small or one-time donations that were "too far away."

Some people mailed milk. April had it sent from North Carolina, always paying for shipping. Several companies specialize in high-tech shipping containers for frozen liquids, and as long as the milk is tightly packed with a coolant, it will stay frozen for a twenty-four-hour journey. Once the package arrives, typically through FedEx or UPS, recipients check the bags, tossing any that are broken or softened.

Frozen milk is defrosted in the refrigerator and then given to the baby with a bottle or supplemental nursing system (SNS). Some parents com-bine milks from different donors, while others use only one milk at a time. Naomi said, "I just used [milk] from one donor at a time, in case there was any reaction or anything. I never noticed that [my baby] did or didn't like any of the milks, but it was always given via SNS at the breast. . . . She never had a bottle, everything has been done at the breast."

Our family decided not to receive milk via shipping because we wanted to meet donors in person. This was based on our desire to have a personal connection to donors and the result of a perhaps fallacious idea that we could learn more about our donors if we met them and their children. As you can see, whatever combination of variables is in play for any one family, the entire practice relies on a matrix of ser-

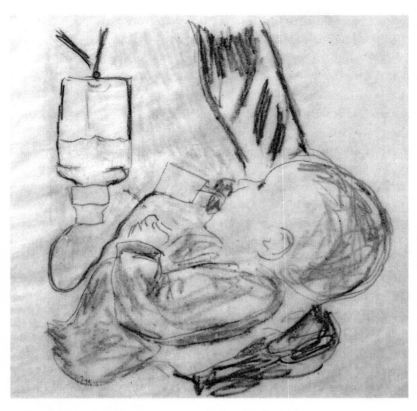

11. Supplemental nursing system at work. Drawing by author.

vices, goods, and technologies. As an anthropologist, I wanted to map this matrix.

I follow the language of my informants, especially when it articulates with theory, so my ears pricked up when Lowry, a donor, described milk distribution as an infrastructure, a current theme in anthropological research. She said, "There is a lot of talk about the banks, but the general consensus is that there should be more of them, and more systematized, so that people can get what they need and it will be safe and there will be a better system for giving it. Look, we need a better system for doing this. . . . We need more of an infrastructure. We need a better system, because a lot more mothers would do this if it were easier, and there are a lot of moms out there who would love to be able to help another mother." Here Lowry views the sharing infrastructure as an externality that could be enhanced but only with improved knowledge and effort.

From Infrastructure to Metastructure

Anthropologists are well positioned to document how infrastructure shapes and is shaped by contemporary life from the ground up. Jonathan Bach, Susan Leigh Star, Julia Elyachar, Daniel Mains, Penny Harvey and Hannah Knox, and Brian Larkin have all used ethnography to trace infrastructures as sites where imaginaries, power, and bodies come together. Nikhil Anand argues that infrastructures are good for investigating matters of interest to anthropologists: the production and maintenance of political authority, how people imagine and ascribe meaning to the world, how infrastructure can operate as a political technology of rule (since it is through the extension and regulation of physical and social infrastructures that biopolitics often works), and how the circulation of goods, at times across great distances, refracts and reproduces inequalities (Anand 2011; Anand et al. 2012).

In their introduction to an issue of *Cultural Anthropology*, Jessica Lockrem and Adonia Lugo (2011) define infrastructures as systems that enable the circulation of goods, knowledge, meaning, people, and power. Larkin (2013) defines infrastructures as material forms that allow for the possibility of exchange over space. Infrastructure is a useful analytic for the distribution patterns associated with many different kinds of entities because it calls attention to the active forging of relationships among materiality, processes, politics, and identity. As a structuring element in any community, infrastructure can go largely unnoticed, at least by some people, but it may be critical to the production of the everyday, especially when basics such as water or electricity are involved. Infrastructures may be accessible only by select people, or spectacular, as when the design, construction, or maintenance of infrastructure is part of a larger political project. Infrastructures may move in and out of visibility as political, economic, or social projects emerge or recede.

Star (1999) explains that the basic characteristic of infrastructure is that it tends, like milk sharing, to be both relational and ecological, making it difficult to examine with traditional ethnographic methods that were developed to examine the lives of people in particular places.

She argues that we need to "scale up" from traditional ethnographic sites to look at infrastructures that engage many hundreds if not many thousands or even millions of people and that can extend across vast geographical areas. The labor- and analysis-intensive craft of qualitative research combined with a historical privileging of single-authored works has never lent itself to an ethnography of thousands, but in focusing on local networks within a global system we can still "surface" relatively quiet voices, identify master narratives, and get at the difference between online and offline activities while also recognizing infrastructural design and practice to identify who is included or excluded, why, and where (Star 1999, 383). So, who can get milk to flow away from or toward themselves, in what quantity, and under what circumstances? What impact does milk sharing have aside from moving milk?

We can examine milk sharing broadly as an "assemblage" or collection of people, technologies, and knowledge joined through distributed agency, as some scholars of science, technology, and society (STS) or material culture have done. This would allow us not only to look at circulation but also to ask about materiality. How might we identify the outlines of the milk infrastructure, taken as matter or as an assemblage? Larkin's (2013, 330) reminder about infrastructural studies is worth quoting at length:

> Discussing an infrastructure is a categorical act. It is a moment of tearing into those heterogeneous networks to define which aspect of which network must be discussed and which parts will be ignored. It recognizes that infrastructures operate on differing levels simultaneously, generating multiple forms of address, and that any particular set of intellectual questions will have to select which of these levels to examine. Infrastructures are not[,] in any positivist sense, simply "out there." The act of defining an infrastructure is a categorizing moment. Taken thoughtfully, it comprises a cultural analytic that highlights the epistemological and political commitments involved in selecting what one sees as infrastructural (and thus causal) and what one leaves out.

To pursue questions about who gets milk, how, and why, as well how subjectivities are produced and performed, I suggest making a rather practical distinction between people and objects that act as prosthetics of human agency. I follow Larkin (2008, 5, 6) in looking at "institution-alized networks that facilitate the flow of goods in a wider cultural as well as physical sense," where infrastructure is the "totality of both technical and cultural systems that create institutionalized structures whereby goods of all sorts circulate." The people then constitute publics that thicken around these forms (De Boeck 2012). (There is a way to think of the lactating body itself as infrastructural, a move that would provide many insights, but I will leave that for now.)

Rendering the milk-sharing infrastructure as an emerging, ever-changing architecture of delivery to a diverse group of users is instructive during a time of intensifying contest and commodification because it points us to larger issues of governance and ideology. One of the first moves in such an analysis is to identify how the very materiality of milk enables and constrains its circulation, value, and meaning.

We both interpret the world and insert ourselves into it by interacting with material culture, or what we call "goods," "things," "commodities," "objects," "products," "artifacts," or even just "stuff."[19] Examining milk as material culture raises both empirical and theoretical questions: What role does milk play in the performance of identity, within practices of social organization, and in shaping subjective experience? How can we delineate the boundaries of milk? What, if any, are the differences between milk in the context of a laboratory versus the substance used by parents (and others) who are pointing at it, intending themselves into the world through it, or using it in identity making?

Studies of material culture can be undertaken through close study of particular objects. A full analysis of milk would consider both physical and semiotic dimensions. We could begin with the construction of value. As material culture, milk, like gold, is expensive, although in May 2015 an ounce of gold was priced at $1,225, while an ounce of milk went for as little as $1.[20] Gold is also, unlike milk, relatively rare, with all of the gold mined since the dawn of civilization fitting into a cube measuring twenty meters per dimension (171,300 tonnes). There are significant differences, but consider these expressions: "it is as good as gold," "he has heart of gold," "she is sitting on a gold mine," "it was a gold-medal performance," and "you've got the golden touch." These expressions point to the superior value we place on the yellow element identified as gold. Sharers routinely refer to breast milk as "white gold" or "liquid gold," where goldness, a quality abstracted from a metal (what Peirce would have referred to as a "qualisign"), stands for that which is coveted, treasured, and valuable and attached to mothers' milk in a move to imbue it with the same.

Like milk, gold was prized long before recorded history. It was one of the first metals used by humans because it occurs in its elemental form (like milk). Dense, shiny, and malleable, it is a good candidate for jewelry, coinage, and other plastic arts. Gold is highly conductive and resists corrosion, which makes it a natural choice for wiring in electronics: cell phones, global positioning devices, computers, and large appliances like televisions, for example, all contain small amounts of gold. Space exploration has also relied on gold: hammered into the thinnest of films, gold reflects dangerous radiation. And it has been used to treat medical conditions. Its malleability and chemical inertness make it good for molding dental crowns. I don't think anyone has overlooked hip-hop culture's use of gold on teeth (to make "fronts" or "grillz") as a symbol of power. A similar move, interpreting the metal metaphorically, as valuable and beautiful, perhaps even divine, underpins the widespread historical and contemporary use of gold in food. And though there are substitutes for gold, its material qualities have led to specialized uses. But still, gold's material versatility and aesthetic character do not completely explain its meaning and wow factor, which is partly a cultural phenomenon.

Milk also has physical characteristics that shape its place in society: breast milk has a flavor and smell. If you want to try it, expect a somewhat nutty and fatty taste that, not surprisingly, will probably remind you of cow's milk. It is sweeter and less tangy than goat's milk. The content and taste of human milk have been shaped during the course of evolutionary history: that humans evolved to like sweet, fatty tastes is no coincidence. But besides the flavor, milk delivers nutrients, water, and antibodies that shift over the course of the day, as the infant ages, with regard to what a mother consumes, and over the course of a feeding.

As a result of these shifts, milk-sharing families may attempt to match one another according to babies' ages, pay attention to diet, or ask questions about when a donor pumps (for example, does a donor pump only after her own baby has nursed (when milk is the fatty hindmilk) or only before (for more watery foremilk), or are pumping sessions done separately from nursing sessions (in which case the milk would be a combination of hind- and foremilk). Some of our donors were vigilant in labeling milk as hindmilk or foremilk or a combination of both, while others practiced a simple pump-and-freeze procedure.

Enabled by pump-and-freeze technology, sharing is a cyborgian pursuit. And it requires space and privacy, all of which can be supported, or not, by policy. Part of the reason the sharing population consists largely of stay-at-home moms is that, for most women, pumping and then storing breast milk at work is a major challenge. Amber, who was a milk donor and later a recipient, works to improve maternity care practices in institutions throughout the state in her capacity as a lactation consultant employed by the Georgia Department of Public Health. She points out that the practice of feeding babies mothers' milk suffers from a combination of physical hurdles and structural inadequacies: "There is a lack of adequate maternity leave, and by that I mean paid maternity leave, and a complete lack of support for public breast feeding. So many moms feel sequestered at home. And many childcare places are not breastfeeding friendly. Then you have to consider that many work places lack the support required for breast pumping or feeding." She continued with examples from her own experience:

> Many of my own friends who have gone back to work didn't last pumping for very long because it is not easy and it is not a break: pumping is work! I have had to pump while at training sessions and I can tell you, it is not fun. You are sitting there with your breasts hooked up to a machine, and a lot of times your body might need a little help from a hand (I have always needed hands on) because not everyone has an easy let down with a machine and a little massage adds a human aspect at least. So a lot of times, you can't eat or do anything else on your "break."

In addition, Amber pointed out that some coworkers may object to breast milk in the work fridge or the sight of a pump.[21]

Store-ability has huge implications for sharing. Most people who mail frozen milk use an overnight service like FedEx and specially packed boxes. If there is a delay in transit, the milk can soften, creating the possibility for bacterial growth. Knowing this potentiality, parents typically discard thawed milk. Milk picked up locally is not nearly as vulnerable to this problem, which is why many families participate only in local shares.

Haylee decided not to ship her milk because she did not want to leave it on the road for pickup; she worried that someone might take it or that the FedEx driver might miss it, leaving it to spoil under the hot Georgia sun. For others it may not make sense to ship—April, for example, only shipped larger amounts from donors whom she already had met face to face. Others, like Margaret, did not want to meet in person at all; she felt it was too personal. Our family decided not to participate in shipping after we had a delivery snafu: we were not at home to sign the documents, and even though the driver brought the package back that evening, some of the bags were soft and dripping.

Like milk, the infrastructure for sharing is both material and immaterial. Star (1999) defines infrastructure as "embedded," sunk into other structures, social arrangements, and technologies. Milk sharing is sunk into an assortment of social arrangements, technologies, and other infrastructures such as pumps (and associated plastics manufacturing and electrical infrastructures), storage tools (freezers, refrigerators, coolers, dry ice, high-tech equipment, plastic bags), shipping systems (FedEx, the U.S. Postal Service, or UPS and high-tech coolants for shipping), roads, digital tools (such as computers, cell phones, fax machines, Internet browsers, Facebook, Internet sites, personal messaging, cameras, email, and other equipment), and medical practices (including but not limited to medical records technology, insurance, and blood tests). Sharing is also predicated on social acceptance and fluency in participating in virtual communities, a competency that has emerged only in the last few years as we have become comfortable interacting through online avatars.

As Harvey and Knox's (2015) study of roads illustrates so clearly, infrastructure is contingent upon an assemblage of technologies (such as civil engineering, physics, and material studies), knowledges (from computers to political science, to international funding instruments, to state policy, and so forth), and social activity (for example, "buy-in" by local populations), and, even if it is discontinuous in places, it enables the flow of goods, acts as a symbol of modernity, and indexes state power (even as that state power is unevenly broadcast, especially in more remote areas). Infrastructure has a literal function (in the case of roads, related to transportation), but additional "goods" (such as the construction of connectivity, nationalism, or the future) are ferried on top. The movement of milk also requires moving "milk" in a variety of registers from material culture to cultural material.

And while technically milk sharing is open to everyone, people may be effectively excluded because they lack access to the Internet, lack time to interact online, and so forth. The digital interface may repel users, like Kiki, who wanted to become a donee but felt overwhelmed with the Facebook page, or Marsha, who wanted to become a donor but did not want to "get involved with the whole online thing." But Marsha did go through her local parents' group since she knew many participants personally, in real life.

Again following Star (1999), sharing becomes more transparent through use: immaterial aspects such as the performance of community values and conventions (such as demonstrating neediness as a donee or exchanging private information offline), discussions of legal standards (which are in fact limited but seem to be on the horizon), mobilizations of medical knowledge (about the benefits or possible dangers of breast milk sharing), and debates over the political directionality of advanced capitalism (especially with regard to thinking of the body "as a cash machine") become easier to see and evaluate over time. And though they do not use these terms participants are hashing out the meanings of human nature, human relationships, and human bodies, all of which impinge upon the shape and character of milk distribution.

Using infrastructure as a theoretical lens is useful because it calls attention to the way that an overall apparatus of distribution is constructed, contested, and maintained by sharers. As infrastructure, milk sharing interacts with larger contexts, has both material and immaterial aspects, and directs milk in different ways. But the apparatus is unusual compared to many projects (such as water, roads, or electrical infrastructures) in that it is neither state nor industry sponsored, nor is its "good" commodified, but also in that people can and in fact must pick and choose among a set of already-existing infrastructures that do not exist primarily for this purpose. To call attention to this infrastructural bricolage, I use the term "metastructure."

Milk sharing requires cobbling together a metastructure, and this metastructure encourages sharers to meet new people.[22] But how does it address and constitute subjects? Breast milk sharers—who, I will argue in the next chapter, constitute a "counternetwork" that coalesces around this metastructure—are subalterns who adhere to values opposed by hegemonic institutions. Even though people posting on social media do not necessarily know one another, there is enough community overlap to maintain a set of principles. The population shifts as parents' needs change (as donors or donees), and there are positions (such as site administrators) that allow people to exert more power than an ordinary seeker or giver of milk, but in most ways there is no final authority figure or hierarchy. And this metastructure is vast. Nobody is in charge, yet it is quite stable and very efficient. So who are these milky moms who offer their white gold to strangers? How well did we, could we, know them?

Romana Caritas

Following the Council of Trent (1545–63), the breast became more sexualized for Western Europeans. Images of Mary breastfeeding became less common. But another trope emerged: the tale of Charity. "Charity," a term of love harkening to the Greek ἀγαπᾶν, "to treat with affectionate regard," might well be applied to milk donation.

Valerius Maximus, the ancient Roman writer, recounted the tale known today as "Roman Charity." Incarcerated for life, the elderly Cimon was denied food by his jailers (to hasten his death). To save him, his daughter Pero gained access to his cell and offered him her breast milk. The guards, impressed with Pero's selflessness, released Cimon from prison.

There are many illustrations of this story, including an early fresco from Pompeii, Italy (artist unknown), dating from the first century. Roman Charity was also taken up by artists in the seventeenth and eighteenth centuries.

There are even contemporary versions, such as *Romana Caritas* (2011) by the Russian artist Max Sauco, known for his work in surrealism and photo manipulation. Many details in Sauco's work are worth commenting on—from the halo and smoke emanating from Cimon to the phallic wooden post engraved with his name, to the nails and the blood dripping from Cimon's feet, to the quantity of milk spilled on the ground. And, unlike in earlier accounts, there seems to be a somewhat erotic dimension.

Sauco's image could be described as a Salvador Dalí–Joel-Peter Witkin mashup. Both of those artists dealt with breast milk. Dalí's *Fountain of Milk Spreading Itself Uselessly on Three Shoes* (1945) references the lactation of Saint Bernard, but the miraculous milk is spent on a parched landscape from a woman atop a pedestal. Witkin created several works

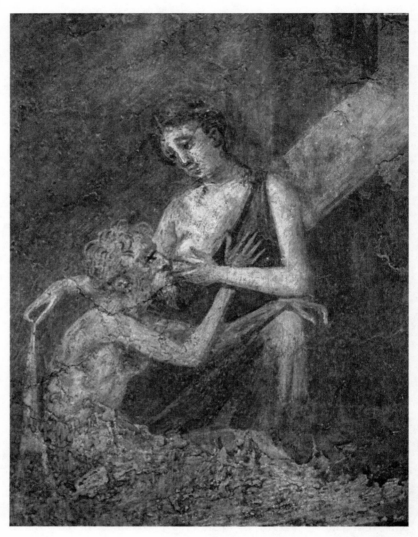

12. Cimon and Pero depicted in a first-century Roman fresco (Pompeii, Italy). Photo by Stefano Bolognini, Wikimedia Commons. https://en.wikipedia.org/wiki/Roman _Charity#/media/File:Affresco_romano_-_Pompei_-_Micon_e_Pero.jpg.

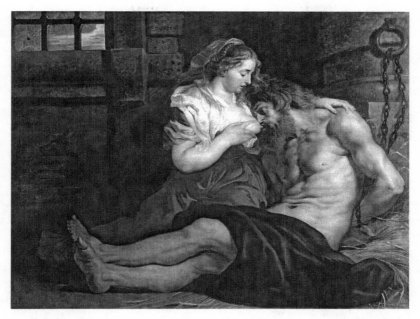

13. Peter Paul Rubens, *Cimon and Pero (Roman Charity)*, c. 1612. Oil on canvas.
https://en.wikipedia.org/wiki/File:Roman_Charity_-_Pieter_Pauwel_Reubens.jpg.

about breastfeeding: *Woman Breastfeeding an Eel* (1980) and *Androgeny Breast Feeding a Fetus* (1981). Both reflect Witkin's surrealist, out-of-bounds style that asks us to examine our own value systems and challenges culturally constructed boundaries between human and animal, life and death, self and other, male and female, and beauty and horror.

The most striking element running throughout these figurations is the depiction of female agency. Pero/Charity is always placed above Cimon, the active partner with the power to pronounce life or death through her gift. On the other hand, it's complicated because Cimon, like any potential donee, has the power to refuse the gift (and everything it entails). As donor Miranda put it,

> I have all this extra [milk] and so I emailed my acupuncturist and tried to give it to them because they had twins and they said, "No thanks!" His wife probably thought it was weird, and I can see that, and I felt a little weird offering. But anyway, I asked Violet, my yoga teacher, if

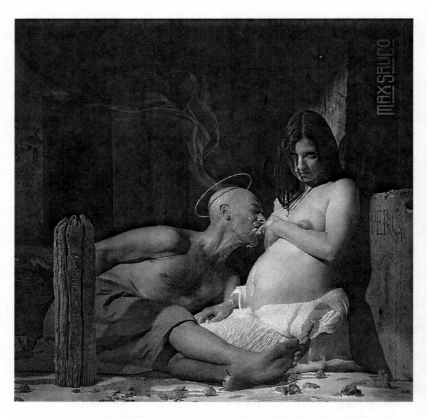

14. Max Sauco, *Romana Caritas*, 2011. Photo-painting. Used with artist's permission.

she wanted it and she was excited and took it and offered free yoga in return, which is pretty great. The thing is that Violet trusts me. She trusts me to treat her baby like I treat my own. I looked on craigslist [a peer-to-peer website for buying and trading] to see what its [sic] going for, and people were charging like $2 or $2.50. I would not do that though; people who are selling it are doing [it] to supplement [their income], but I don't need that, it's not worth it, I can't see doing it because what I get is a sense of gratification. Giving her my milk is a real privilege. She keeps thanking me, but it's really my honor to help her baby with his well-being. It is a privilege that she trusts me. It's very rewarding. And I take that privilege seriously. It's personal. When you sell it, it's not voluntary, giving it is important. If I sold it, I would feel like a milk cow. And not to disparage those who chose to do that—because maybe it allows her to have some income to stay home with her baby and that's great—and maybe I get "paid" by the yoga, but I would do it anyway . . . and it's a nice trade, but it is totally outside the market. I'm a communist! But I would donate to a bank or stranger too. Not sell it. If Violet offered me money I would be pissed!

Other donors explained how they felt empowered by making and giving milk and by the trust placed in them by donees. Giving milk is not only a form of charity; it is a powerful act and even, as Giles (2010) has suggested in another context, a form of self-care.

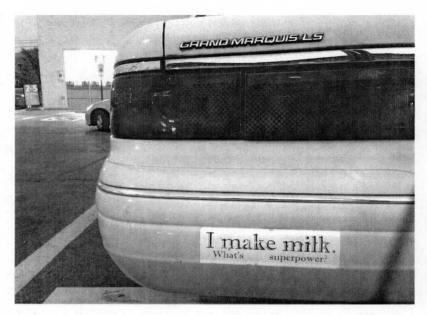

15. "I make milk. What's your superpower?," 2014. Bumper sticker. Photo by James Bielo. Used with permission.

2   A Complicated Gift

Effie, who is white and middle class, lives in her own single-family home with her husband and two kids in a suburban neighborhood. She is active in the local La Leche League community and would like to eventually join the LLL leadership. She is Christian, patriotic, and pro-military. She eats organic foods, avoids alcohol and caffeine, uses cloth diapers, and is suspicious of vaccines. She homeschools her children and practices baby-led "attachment parenting," which means following the principles of childrearing promoted by the best-selling author and pediatrician William Sears. This style of childrearing asks a lot of mothers and fathers.

In addition to helping me find other donors, Effie was a regular donor to our family. She was an overproducer, making more milk than her baby could consume, and she was a self-proclaimed lactivist, believing wholeheartedly that all babies should be fed breast milk if possible. We were thrilled to find each other.

Over and above the milk itself Effie viewed donation as community making. When I picked up the milk, it was a social event. We visited in the southern sense of the word, which meant that she invited me in and gave me food and drink. I saw the public parts of her house. We talked about our children's latest accomplishments, our husbands, baby-proofing our houses, and day-to-day activities. It was a time for learning about each other while our kids played.

I was careful not to make pointed or sarcastic comments about religion or politics. This was partly because it is considered unseemly to discuss politics or religion with acquaintances in many parts of the South, and Effie never asked me about my religious beliefs or political leanings. But everyone gets the basics (I am nonreligious and left leaning) according to what is said, since we are of course always telling people who we are—ethnically, religiously, economically, educationally, politically, and otherwise—through how we talk, regardless of the content of our conversation. We did, on the other hand, discuss breast milk, the pharmaceutical industry, the politics of formula, public education, and how baby products like diapers, car seats, and bottles are marketed. We agreed that milk sharing was doing an "end run" around for-profit formula companies. She stopped donating only when she became pregnant with her third child.

Counternetwork

This chapter is devoted to exploring the stories of women who, like Effie, are donors. Who are these "milky moms"? Why do they do it? What conditions make donating possible? What does the moral economy of gifting milk look like? What are the political implications? How do people interact with the metastructure (which can, as I suggested in chapter one, be cleaved from the network of people who coalesce around it)?

Sharers coalesce around a metastructure as they question, resist, selectively follow, and bypass institutional authority. Some donors and donees are connected through friends, breastfeeding groups, doulas, midwives, or lactation consultants, but most donors I worked with, those who donated to our family and those I interviewed, do not know one another.

One way to conceptualize this group is as a public. In academic investigations of this concept one work of special note is Jürgen Habermas's ([1962] 1989) on the historicity of the public sphere, where "public" is built upon ideals of equality, rational discourse, and participation in civic space. Subsequent refinements have advanced how such a public is thought to operate.

In her critique of Habermas's public Nancy Fraser (1992) wields a feminist sensibility to outline the emergence of postbourgeois, subaltern "counterpublics," which form their own interest groups. Fraser argues that recognizing a multiplicity of counterpublics whose members and thus voices are subordinated by dominant groups better captures a promise for participatory democracy; subaltern counterpublics can produce counterdiscourses that address and request a response from dominant public discourse.

Michael Warner (2002) describes publics as modern relations among strangers similarly interpolated. These stranger publics are imagined in advance, activated by the uptake of text, and cease to exist when attention is no longer predicated (88). While ephemeral, they contribute to the warp and weft of the social fabric. Counterpublics are those publics that maintain an awareness of subordination with regard to ideas, genre, and modes of address, with participants acknowledging power relationships through their participation in counterpublic discourse; a counterpublic is identified not just through oppositional politics but also through the nonconformist nature of its intervention, in which "the discourse that constitutes it is not merely a different or alternative idiom, but one that in other contexts would be regarded with hostility or with a sense of indecorousness" (119). You can see how counterpublic dissent may proceed through awkward confrontations and hostile encounters, but even outside of oppositional discourse it is a "politics of refusal" enacted by those whose modes of argument step outside of the frame of established debate altogether (Harvey and Knox 2015, 172).

In responding to a hegemonic "breast milk is best" narrative, sharers can be understood as constituting a powerful, and empowering, counterpublic. But to highlight the enactment of a politics of refusal by people connected through a metastructure, I would suggest using the term "counternetwork." This counternetwork (the set of sharers participating at any one time) is configured against hegemonic norms for baby nourishment (breasts, official banks, and formula), implicitly critiquing medical and pharmaceutical policy. Though people are brought together in uneven, and even stochastic ways, those of like minds about feeding babies, but not necessarily other issues, work together, adding new textures to a body politic.

Because the circulation of milk takes place in particular spaces, at particular times, we can track it ethnographically. The boundaries defining the metastructure are fuzzy because ideas about what makes a good donor or whose milk is most sharable are constantly being (re)negotiated. Can the donor consume meat, alcohol, caffeine, or sleeping pills? What about spicy food? Should milk be commodified? With whom should you, as a donor, share milk? Is it better to give your milk to a premature baby, the first person to ask, or to a baby with special needs, or is it better to sell it to someone for an art project? Should colostrum cost more or be held back for special circumstances? Is it acceptable to donate only foremilk? A bigger question concerns who polices these values: there is no center or authority in this counternetwork. It is self-policing. Sprawling. Rhizomatic. Horizontal.

To get at milk sharing we should take it as historically sited, as an *event*, emerging, extending in time and space, refracting cultural, political, and economic dynamics, and then disappearing. This approach encourages us to attend to the circumstances that enable or discourage milk sharing as a process that interacts with us. Milk means something, but milk sharing "does things," to riff on J. L. Austin's (1962) *How to Do Things with Words*, which argues that linguistic utterances not only have meanings but also consequences, such as engendering particular social relationships.

Configuration

Donors I spoke with highlighted how sharing entails and is entailed by political-economic, cultural, and technological configurations that shape the counternetwork within which identities, desires, and relationships are enacted. The circulation of milk is contingent upon intersecting values promoted by both official and grassroots community organizations. Such values include the virtues of breast milk, laws about milk exchange, and a drive for commodification by for-profit companies (discussed more in chapter five) that are pushing against donation circuits as the practice becomes better known.

As construed by many sharers, "white gold" operates as a mirror image to formulas attempting simulate and sell milk to mothers under the logic of capitalism. To produce milk oneself is itself empowering, and having excess to give to another baby is "fulfilling," "gratifying," an "honor," a way to "pay it forward," and understood as "giving back to the community." Meanwhile mothers discuss risk and the ethics of commodification.

Interestingly there are few laws about breast milk. Forty-nine states, including Georgia, have laws that specifically protect the right of women to breastfeed in any public location, but only three states (New York, California, and Texas) have laws related to the procurement, processing, distribution, or use of human milk (but they pertain to milk moving through a licensed milk bank). According to the legal scholar Stephanie Dawson David (2011), human milk is not included under the National Organ Transplant Act of 1984 (which makes the selling of human organs a federal crime), and many states exclude "replenishable" or "self-replicating" body fluids and tissues (such as milk, hair, and sperm) from the scope of laws prohibiting the sale of bodily materials.

So even though sharers often claimed that "selling milk was illegal," the fact is that under current laws breast milk is treated more like a food than a bodily fluid; buying and selling it is perfectly legal. David (2011), along with others who recognize that current laws offer little protection to buyers who may be harmed by milk bought on informal markets, calls for adopting regulations governing the sale, processing, and shipment of human milk, particularly with regard to impersonal and informal sales, to better ensure the health and safety of children in these transactions. But even if laws with these provisions were passed, they would not apply to milk circulated as gifts.

Although women could make several hundred dollars or more per month selling milk, inside the counternetwork there is a moral measuring of recipients that affects pricing and distribution. For example, Margaret discovered at a support meeting that body builders were buying local milk. A woman in her group was having financial difficulties and asked the others if "it would make her a bad person" if she sold her milk to body builders instead of donating to a needy baby. A few moms admitted that they had already been doing this to contribute to family finances, but most of the others argued, "No way, milk is for babies."

Margaret's comments highlight the hierarchy of need that structures the distribution of milk, with mothers who try and fail but who want to breastfeed being viewed as most deserving and those who choose not to breastfeed because of the work involved being viewed as less deserving. The presence on listservs of offers to donate milk that specify a desire to help a baby with special needs or a premature baby index the tacit rules of donate-ability. Body builders who want milk for its supposed role in muscle growth or men who want it to satisfy a sexual fetish are typically the last to be served (and in following an imagined supply gap, offers to sell milk to men are often accompanied by higher pricing).

Reflecting this hierarchy of need, Chrissy, a Human Milk for Human

Babies site administrator, was explicit about HM4HB aims when she told me in an interview that "our mission is to make sharing commonplace and normal. Moms make informed decisions, both donors and recipients. It is a free choice. But BMS [breast milk sharing] is gaining popularity, especially in the natural birthing community. And many women want to breastfeed but can't, so others step in." HM4HB had its fourth birthday in 2014, and when asked what changes she had observed, Chrissy explained that she had seen the community grow rapidly. When she started there were seven hundred people on the page; by 2014 there were more than twenty-four hundred. The number fluctuates as babies and moms come and go, but there has been a tremendous increase in activity.

The configuration is shaped by technological opportunities and constraints, as well as member participation. Georgia is one of the few states with both a public and a closed group. Many persons expressed privacy concerns to Chrissy, so she started the closed page as an alternative. By 2014 the closed page had about a thousand members. She also expressed concerns about how the architecture of the site was becoming a major issue:

> When Facebook modified their algorithm, things changed. So, I can do a repost, and it used to be that a repost would go to all the people that frequently "like" the page, but now, reposts only go to about 10% at a time. So that's a problem. I mean the whole plan is to make it easy and visible; with the closed group, members control what they see and customize their feeds. So, we are still tweaking and experimenting to find the best way to do this. And why? Because as women and mothers, we have so many options, and so many things that divide us: from birthing, to what kind of diapers to use, to how you parent, but with breast milk sharing, all those differences are put aside. We present a unified front. It is just moms helping moms, or babies who have lost a mother. Or grandparents who suddenly find themselves caring for an infant. Or surrogate fathers. Or adoptive parents. This allows us to come together. It really isn't just a bunch of creepers out there. These are people with good intentions. It really is all about feeding babies.

We can imagine a sharing community functioning (just not as quickly, widely, or effectively) without Facebook group sites or MilkShare, but none of this would be happening without the pump—the machine that cleaves breastfeeding from breast milk and makes it possible to feed a baby breast milk without the presence of a breast. Pumping allows women to extract milk and to save it for later, to give it away, or to sell it. Guinness World Records, an organization that keeps track of human accomplishments, reports that Alyse Ogletree of Argyle, Texas, used pump technology to donate 53,081 ounces of milk to the Mothers' Milk Bank of north Texas, giving her the record as Biggest Milk Donor. Perhaps this is not that surprising, given the social value placed on breastfeeding as essential to a woman's performance as a mother. Those who breastfeed (and by extension those who donate milk) can lay claim to being better women and mothers (Stearns 2010).

Until the 1990s electric breast pumps (developed for hospitals) were unavailable for home use. Today women use hand or electric pumps, even renting or buying "hospital-grade" models secondhand. Valerie explained, "If a baby cannot latch on, moms pump. Or if their baby is in NICU, they pump so that they'll be ready when the baby comes home. But pumping has different rules. For one thing, when you nurse, the baby stops when he's full. But with a pump, you pump until there is no more, and it's more than the baby would take, so you are pumping more than you need. And when you have too much, there are really only two options. You can give it away to someone who cannot furnish enough, or can't furnish any! Or dump it down the sink. And that is just wasteful." But, as Helen explained, "Pumping is a chore! Hooking up your bosoms to a machine and then letting the machine go to town? You feel like a cow! But people do it, and they do it with love when it is for their baby."

Ancient Greeks used a ceramic guttus, both to empty the breast and feed the infant, before the Romans invented glass milk-extractors sucked by the mother herself. Devices in the form of a smoking pipe became widespread in the seventeenth century, and in the nineteenth century vessels sucked both by mother and infant were developed to facilitate breastfeeding for preterm infants (Obladen 2012). Orwell Needham applied for a U.S. patent for his breast pump in 1854. It has not changed that much since then.

Women commented on the clunky, even "medieval" nature of pump

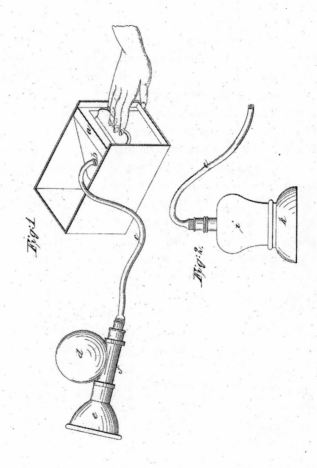

16. Design for breast milk pump as sketched in patent application by
Orwell Needham. http://www.google.com/patents/US11135.

design. "My husband," donor Kristin pointed out, "is not one to point out gender inequalities. I mean he took a women's studies class in college and stuff like that, but he is not really a feminist, but even he was like 'that pump is crazy!' If those were for men, they would be portable and streamlined. When I started pumping, I heard that there was some competition at MIT or somewhere to make a better pump, but I am still waiting for that." I suspect that few engineering resources will be devoted to pump improvements until there is big money to be made. And electric pumps, medieval as they may be, are effective as is.

Mara told me, "I was paranoid about not having enough milk for my baby, and I was working, I mean I am a teacher, so I was pumping like crazy, like thirty ounces a day and freezing it. Pretty soon I had filled up the freezer, but we realized that there was no way the baby was going to go through all of it. And my wife also had an oversupply, and so we starting donating. After all, it is 'liquid gold!'"

The pump, unwieldy as it is, is important to those who work. Some donors, like Murial, can arrange their work to fit their pumping needs. "As the mother of a six-month-old," she said, "I have to pump when I travel. And I travel a lot. But I always call ahead to the airports where I am making a connection to ensure they have a family bathroom where I can do it. If they don't, and not all of them do, I reroute my flight so that I get a connection in a place that has a family room. I am just not going to do it in the bathroom on the plane!" But some mothers find pumping at work extremely challenging or even impossible.

Even stay-at-home mothers pump so they can have time away (when a babysitter can bottle-feed the baby). Some pump when breastfeeding is not possible due to poor latching, maternal medication or surgery, or infant illness. Pumping and storing may allow a nonlactating partner to feed a child using a supplemental nursing system or bottle. Some mothers generate a stash as a kind of "emotional insurance," as one donor put it. Others may not like to breastfeed in public, or at all. Those who have experienced sexual trauma may find breastfeeding upsetting and opt to pump and bottle-feed instead. Others pump when engorged but unable to nurse or when using formula. Sidney explained to me that she always breastfed her baby, enjoyed it, and had an easy time with it because "Haley was a good baby, a good nurser, but I always pumped at night and gave her formula instead because she slept longer like that. If I nursed her, she would wake up every two or three hours."

Cindy Stearns's (2010) analysis of the way pumps are named and advertised describes a cultural matrix in which breastfeeding, or at least feeding a baby breast milk, is essential to performing motherhood. Pump marketers take advantage of the idea that breastfeeding is ideal, natural, and pure, using names like the Ameda Purely Yours Breast Pump or Dr. Brown's Natural Flow Electric Breast Pump with "natural" feeding bottles. But there is nothing "natural" about pumping, which is why lactation consultants are hired to teach new mothers how to do it. In fact, as mothers pointed out, while it can be easy and fast, pumping can also be labor intensive, frustrating, and stressful.

Risks

The same forces—technology, modernity, work policy, and so forth—that brought us the modern pump brought us problems with breast milk. Erin, whose daughter was supplied through donations, had to laugh a little about her own preoccupation with pumped breast milk: "Hannah only had breast milk until she was ten months old, and then we took a trip and didn't have any, so we used formula. We were visiting friends, two gay guys that had adopted two kids, and they had given them formula. Harvey was ribbing us about how we were down on formula. He thought formula was fine and he was kidding us and saying, like an ad tagline, 'baby formula kills.'" But formula, like milk, does have risks, and the milk versus formula question is not a simple one.

For one thing persistent organic pollutants (POPS), which include such scary-sounding compounds as polychlorinated dibenzo-*p*-dioxins (PCDDS), polychlorinated dibenzofurans (PCDFS), polychlorinated biphenyls (PCBS), and organochlorine pesticides (like DDT) tend to accumulate in the food chain over time, with breast milk and breast milk–fed infants at the end of the chain (Mead 2008). Since 1951 DDT and its metabolites have been reported in essentially all breast milk tested worldwide, with additional chemicals showing up since then (including banned POPS). What happens is that lipophilic chemicals (most of which come in through the mother's diet) are stored in body fat over a lifetime, and when that tissue is mobilized to make milk, the body transmits a portion of her (possibly substantial) stores of environmental contaminants to her baby. *Advances in Neonatal Care* reported (Jorrisen 2007) that on average, a nursling receives fifty times (per kilogram of body weight) the daily PCB intake of adults and that breastfed infants are predicted to have cumulative PCB exposure up to 18 percent higher than those of formula-fed infants, depending on the duration of breastfeeding, yet the analysis of research on breast milk exposure indicates that despite the measurably higher PCB loads, breastfed children continue to fare better than their formula-fed peers.

Not only POPs but dangerous metals like lead and mercury, which also accumulate in the body, can contaminate breast milk. However, these metals have been detected in even higher concentrations in commercial formula, and the (competing) protective effects of breast milk may outweigh the potential harm generated by heavy metal contamination.

Looking at the intersection of gender, reproduction, and environmental degradation, Maia Boswel-Penc's (2006) *Tainted Milk* examines the complex relationship between the politics of feminist and environmentalist groups and the lack of public awareness in the United States about the presence of chemical toxins in what is supposed to be an unadulterated substance. The relative public silence about this issue has meant that policy responses to environmental pollutants linked to contaminated milk have been minimal (in Sweden, as a point of comparison, policy limiting pesticide and fire retardant use have made the environment healthier for both infants and adults). While some environmental activists have been reluctant to worry aloud about milk contamination lest it discourage women who do breastfeed from continuing to do so, some feminists have been reluctant to promote breastfeeding as a biologically endowed feature of motherhood because they argue it reproduces an essentialist notion of gender.

And then there are the risks associated with sharing. Shanna, a donor who temporarily turned to donated milk when she was on medication to treat a persistent case of thrush, recognized that the stakes for a donee family are different than for the donor:

> The whole donor-donee thing is interesting. I mean back in the day
> wet nurses fed babies. So, it has been going on forever, but in a dif-

ferent format. Now there is a step in between. But donating is easy. It is not a big deal[.] But being a donee? Now, that's a big deal. You have to be careful: What has this woman been eating and drinking? How does she treat her body? What is her lifestyle? Does she have any weird germs? Any bonehead can give, but you have to be brave and savvy to receive. It is like blood! At a milk bank, there are checks. And I do not have a clue about that side yet—I mean how do you gently ask about someone's HIV status or whether they have ever had syphilis? I mean are you like: "Do you have the clap? 'Cuz, if you do, I don't want your milk!'" I mean you don't want to alienate or insult someone who is about to give you a precious gift. That's pretty tricky. Being a receiver is a WAYYY bigger deal.

Shanna is right: issues of disease and contamination are real. Breast milk can carry HIV, hepatitis, and other diseases. Almost every donor we contacted in 2010 provided medical records for us. At times the records had been generated during the pregnancy, while at other times women made appointments with a health care provider to get additional tests. I noticed in the way people were responding to us that over time (as the practice seems to be growing) more sharers seemed to be participating in higher-risk situations. Some donors we contacted in 2012, for example, were not willing to have tests or to disclose medical information. One plainly stated that the request for information was too intrusive. Another told us that her medical information was private, and she was uncomfortable sharing it. Others did not have time to acquire records or to take tests. Some explained that no one else had made these requests and that they would rather look for an easier exchange, one that did not require documentation.

And then there is the possibility of contamination. Research on donor milk contamination has become more vigorous in the last decade. An article in *Pediatrics* on microbial contamination of breast milk purchased on the Internet, cited in popular media like the *New York Times*, reported that an analysis of a cross-sectional sample (n = 101) of milk purchased from an online breast milk sharing website, when compared to milk bank samples (n = 20), "exhibited high overall bacterial growth and frequent contamination with pathogenic bacteria, reflecting poor collection, storage, or shipping practices," and the authors concluded that "infants consuming this milk are at risk for negative outcomes, particularly if born preterm or . . . medically compromised" (Keim et al. 2013, e1227).

Keim et al.'s (2013) study was designed to compare the potential for milk bought online versus unpasteurized samples from milk banks to cause infectious disease. Analysis of samples in each set showed that milk bought anonymously online contained gram-negative, coliform, and streptococcus bacteria (the milk bank samples also contained these bacteria, though not salmonella, but at much smaller levels). Studies have also found dangerous contamination in formula (see Langreth and Nussbaum 2011). For breast milk samples bought online, each additional day in transit was associated with an increase in bacterial count. But what long- and short-term risks do these microbe loads represent?

In a separate study, Keim and her team tested 102 samples of milk purchased from online sources and found that 10 samples contained a level of bovine DNA consistent with human milk mixed with at least 10 percent cow's milk, which could be problematic for infants with allergies or intolerance. Adulteration (with cow's milk, formula, or something else) could be accidental or deliberate, but as the authors point out, "selling rather than donating milk involves a monetary exchange, which may increase numerous risks, similar to those documented for how paying blood donors increases the likelihood of infectious disease markers in the blood supply" (Keim et al. 2015, 4).

However, this contamination study was set up only to approximate "real-life transactions." Sellers were sent a standard email inquiry expressing interest in buying a small quantity of milk. Communications were confined to the transaction, and all correspondence ceased if the seller asked about a recipient infant or insisted on telephone or in-person communication (57 out of 495 inquiries). Email, PayPal address, and delivery address were anonymous. No instructions were given about shipping methods.

In related research, titled "Breast Milk Sharing via the Internet," Keim and her team analyzed postings by sharers to discover how participants communicate about health and safety risks (Keim et al. 2014). They found that few donor postings reflected measures that could reduce risk (e.g., good hygiene, specifics about disease screenings, abstaining from substances). And 90 percent of the recipients did not specify health or safety practices. Such data led the team to conclude that a lack of communication may exacerbate the health risks for recipient infants, especially those at increased risk.

This study (Keim et al. 2014) is provocative, but even the authors admit that offline activity was unavailable to them. In my experience this offline activity is where many personal questions related to health, hygiene, disease, diet, and so forth would be asked and answered. And one of the most important aspects of the sharing relationship as advanced by network members and sites like MilkShare is having good communication between participants. What Keim's study seems to miss is the tacit expectation that donors enter into these discussions privately because some information is not meant for public consumption. Some information is exchanged on a need-to-know basis: for example, if a recipient had a breast surgery that went horribly wrong and she now cannot breastfeed, that may be private. If a donor takes a psychotropic pill for postpartum depression, she may reveal this privately.

Echoing my own observations, Stuebe, Gribble, and Palmquist (2014) argue that the design of Keim et al.'s research—with its anonymous purchase, no-questions-asked format and lack of packaging requirements for shipping—is unlikely to be representative of real parents seeking milk, for several reasons: (1) the vast majority of parents seeking milk, 96 percent in one analysis, use only sites that promote donation (not sales); (2) the authors did not screen donors, whereas real parents typically do; and (3) milk-gifting sites encourage local delivery over shipping, which would reduce the risk of microbial growth during poorly designed transit, resulting in an analysis of a "worst-case scenario" for milk sharing.

Research on milk samples from the kind of sharing I have been describing in these chapters is needed, as is research on the extent to which microbes represent dangers to most babies receiving donor milk (in contrast to those especially vulnerable infants we might typically find in a NICU). Keim et al.'s study makes me wonder to what extent milk routinely expressed, frozen, bottled, and then given by mothers to their own children across the entire population would not present the same set of microbes. Most of the milk our family received, well over twenty-five thousand ounces, was initially pumped and frozen for someone's own child.

Keim et al. (2013, e1228) suggest that "informal sharing" is actively hazardous. I would also note that the use of the term "informal" to describe sharing outside of governmental and institutional surveillance carries a strong implication of illegitimacy as compared to the unmarked category of milk bank exchanges, which we must assume constitute formal (and thus legitimate) exchanges. As a solution to the milk supply gap, Keim et al. (2013, e1227) suggest that "lactation support services could begin to address the milk supply gap for women who want to feed their child human milk but cannot [themselves] meet the baby's needs." And while such support could undoubtedly help in many cases, there are parents (like my husband and myself) who will never produce breast milk in sufficient quantities, or maybe not at all, no matter how much lactation support they receive. Here I am thinking of women who foster or adopt, or those who have had mastectomies or breast reductions, or who have other physical conditions (such as polycystic ovaries or hypo-thyroidism) that limit milk production, not to mention male and trans-gendered parents who may want to give their children breast milk but cannot themselves produce it.

So far I have been unable to locate even one example of a child sick-ened by breast milk donated through a local network, or even from milk sold through an online forum. Not to jinx it, but milk sharing seems to be working well. Risky as it may be from a certain perspective, it seems to have a better safety record than banks or formula. Many I spoke with certainly see it this way.

Science says sharing is risky, but then "so is not giving your baby breast milk," as Mara put it and as the "breast milk is best" campaign would have us believe. And the sharing community does recognize risk but views potential problems as manageable and that shared breast milk is worth the risk. But as Karleen Gribble (2014) has pointed out in an early published work on milk gifting (not sales) based on written ques-tionnaires administered to donors and recipients recruited via Facebook, risk mitigation can be improved; for example, donors could be better trained in hygienic expression, and health care providers could be trained to discuss risk mitigation with peer sharers. As McKenna commented, "a lot of people ask about moms who do this, about their honesty and safety, but most people are really honest and when asked, are forthcoming. They have nothing to lose by saying, 'Yeah, I have a glass of wine sometimes,' or 'I do [eat] dairy' and then people can decide whether it is for them." Donors described all kinds of questions based on variables selected to manage risk: Do you have an organic diet? Are you gluten free? Have you been around pets? Do you take vitamins?

Risk management is highly individuated. Stephanie was able to exclusively breastfeed her son for the first six months and then kept nursing him up to about eighteen months. She recounted,

> When he was about four or five months old, he and I were diagnosed with a milk-soy allergy and so I went on a soy- and dairy-free diet. But I am a working mother, so I was pumping at work, and I had built up quite a supply—but since I went dairy- and soy-free, and we both felt better, I did not want to give him the dairy and soy diet milk. So it was just there in my freezer. But I held on to it for a while, because you know, I guess I needed a security blanket. I had a big stash that I could use in a real emergency.

She never did need the milk from when she was eating dairy and soy, but she found a recipient for it who never asked if she was dairy free.

Many moms I spoke with told me they had been anxious about running out of milk and had, especially in the beginning of their child's life, pumped frequently but then found they didn't need it. Laura reached out through her local Facebook group when she felt confident that her baby would not need her frozen supply. She described the group as "a natural, positive parenting group." She wrote in a Facebook posting that she had milk to donate and then described herself: "I do not smoke or drink, and I am healthy." She explained,

> I just listed a few basics. And there was a mom, Gayle, in our group who had a preemie, and the baby was going to be in the NICU for two or three months. So he was very premature. And she was having trouble getting her supply up, which happens when you are not with the baby all the time. I know that happened to me when I had to go back to work. And anyway, she was going to use the milk for the baby

in the NICU. She came and picked it up here and took it to the hospital where she kept it. We live in the same town, so we had some friendship connections, I mean, our kids were born in the same hospital and we had the same midwife, so our circles were entwined, but I had never actually met her or anything before this.

She expressed surprised that Gayle didn't ask her for medical records:

I am aware that certain things can pass through. We did have a superficial Q and A session where she asked me about smoking and drinking, and general health and medication. I told her that I had pets—we have two dogs—I am not sure why people want to know that, but I had seen other people mention that, so I mentioned it to her. She asked me a lot of questions about my process—she wanted to know when it was frozen and how it was frozen, and whether or not it had ever been thawed out—so she was definitely concerned with freshness. I told her that I had used a double electric pump and that I had frozen it in a deep freezer immediately and that it had been in there ever since. So, I am not sure how people decide what is good. I mean, what effect does having pets have? I chose to volunteer that information based on what I had seen other people say because I didn't really know what to say, but I was happy to answer all of her questions. All told, I gave her about 150 ounces.

Other donors reported similar experiences with donees who either did not care or did not know to ask about their donors' health status. Sarah told me,

It occurred to me to talk to her about health issues, so I went to my lactation consultant, Jaye, and she was like "I should really find out about this," and she went and found a long questionnaire for me, and I filled it out and gave it to Kelley, the donee, mainly because I had to have a blood transfusion after my C-section. And I knew that was the only risk because I am very healthy generally. But she did not ask for anything, and she seemed very appreciative that I had filled out these questions for her. So, we met a bunch of times and talked about hanging out—we never did, you know you get so busy with a baby—but it was a really friendly and enjoyable acquaintance. So she knew me, and we did have friends in common.

But, really I got involved because I just felt so lucky that it was going well for me, and I could make that choice because I had time to pump, and I realize that not everyone does—it was an opportunity for me to help, and it seemed so easy. I loved it. I mean I just hook up to a pump and watch a show, and just like that, I am helping someone else!

Donating like this is very personal and because of that, it is very safe, and it is also about the community helping each other. Sure, you can go to a bank and get milk that has been mixed together and tested and all of that stuff but it's not the same. Here you can feel really good: you know the person and her baby!

Not everyone can or wants to meet a sharing partner in person. Some donors felt that the relationship would be too charged. Mara explained,

I never met the donees. I let my partner deal with that because it is very emotional. I mean it is a lot of hard work: I was pumping every time I had a free second because I was so concerned about the baby, and I do want to share it, and I was so happy to be able to do that. I was so proud to be feeding three kids but at the same time, I mean, it is a body fluid. It is part of me and I am passing it on. It is like giving away a piece of yourself. There is an intimacy to it. It's a complicated gift.

The value of community building and developing personal relationships and trust inside the network is not to be underestimated. Since most shares are local, the knowledge that develops is reminiscent of what Julia Elyachar (2010) describes as "secrets of the trade," which are not the property of individuals but emanate from the conduits through which actors emerge. These "secrets," like trading photos of babies, exchanging medical documentation, asking about a person from a shared midwife, visiting someone in their home, or knowing someone virtually on a parenting group website, are missing from scientific studies of milk sharing. To successfully enter the counternetwork, donees and donors must pick up tacit knowledge of what to expect and how to ask questions in an appropriate way. Donors expect to learn why parents need milk. And donees like Amy, who needed milk because breast reduction surgery resulted in a low supply, always sent Sarah, her donor, pictures of the baby, saying, "Look at those rolls!" We also sent our donors photos of our children and kept in touch with them about their progress.

Politics of Refusal

Mothers often appealed to forms of knowledge making outside of rational scientific methods, such as instinct and feelings of trust, to decide with whom to share. These other forms of being or knowing underpin identities enacted in a relational, counternetworked practice. While the hegemony of "breast is best" shapes the larger context, there are all kinds of idiosyncratic reasons women get involved, at times paying no heed whatsoever to scientific or institutional authorities. Donors share to "pay it forward," to cope, to advance a political agenda, or to perform friendship or kinship.

Miranda said she was "fortunate enough to exclusively breastfeed my son until introducing solids, but I pumped every day and donated to a friend with supply problems." Sarah not only donated to strangers-who-became-acquaintances but also cross-nursed babies of two friends (and they nursed her own son). Mara donated to four anonymous donees but also had three friends who had babies around the same time she did, so she pumped for them as a supplement. "One anonymous donee," Mara explained, "asked for a lot of information, but the others did not ask for anything. I had disclosed that I take an asthma medication to a friend and she was like if 'it's good enough for your baby it's good enough for mine'! Another friend said, kind of joking, 'you're not taking any heavy drugs or anything are you?'"

This last remark goes to the unspoken trust operating between friends or family. Donees often assumed that a friend or sister would not harm a child by doling out "bad" milk by failing to disclose medication (legal or illegal), drinks (coffee or alcohol), or disease. Frankly it did not even cross my mind to ask my sister for medical records or tests. Danielle explained that when her sister got pregnant and had a baby at eighteen, the baby was adopted by another family, and at the same time her cousin Pamela also had a baby. Pamela pumped and shipped milk to the family who adopted the baby. "It was all in the family, it was a full circle," she said.

For others, sharing helped them "to cope" with loss or grief. Katherine told me, "I had never even heard of this before we (she and I) started doing it, but since then I had another friend who became a donor. But her case was tragic. She had a great pregnancy, but when she gave birth, the baby was stillborn, and of course, it was really traumatic. But instead of taking medicine to stop her milk from coming in, she let it come. And she pumped for about five or six weeks, and donated the milk. It was just really sad, but that is something she did to help cope with it."

Others, like McKenna, said donating helped them cope with grief in the way that organ donation may feel therapeutic. McKenna moved to Georgia because her military husband was stationed here. McKenna, a stay-at-home mom to two young children, also works as a midwife. She raises goats, chickens, and vegetables and sells beauty products. Because she is deeply involved with the birthing and women's community, she could help my family find donors. When I explained why I was conducting interviews, she wanted to participate because she thought this book was a "great idea because a lot of people do not even know that sharing is an option." I had to agree; whenever I told friends what we were doing, they were at least surprised, often curious, and at times more than a little skeptical.

McKenna's participation started out with allo-nursing with a friend. "I got involved with this," she explained, "because my daughter, Hanna, had been nursed by friend of mine, and so she became ever more near and dear to my heart because this experience was just so super special, and now we have an even closer relationship. Because it is just such a special gift. It's from your heart, from your body." But her introduction to more intensive milk sharing was unanticipated, the result of a connection to an awful situation:

Then, I really got involved in being a regular donor. My donee was a close friend, and after she gave birth she was in a car accident. Well, I say she was in a car accident, but really [what] she had was an undiagnosed heart issue. She had noticed something was wrong but at the time, it was just so close to the baby being born, that her doctor attributed it to the pregnancy. Then, about three or four months after giving birth, she was dropping off her dad at the airport and she got pulled over. That made her heart race, you know, the sirens and everything, which would make anyone's heart race, and the stress was just too much. And she ended up pulling over, of course, and the officer didn't know what was going on. How could he have known? But anyway, when he got out of his car, she fell over and ended up hitting the gas and driving her car over to the other side of the road into oncoming traffic. He just thought she was resisting arrest or trying to escape and he went back to his car and called it in and waited for back up, really just doing his job, he did what he thought he needed to do. But all that time, she was having a heart attack. So, by the time they got to her it was really too late. When they called me, she was still alive, but only by life support, so she did not make it. I was just called in to say goodbye.

She was a close friend; she had even been at my birth. So, I guess [donating] was my mission, or maybe just my way of coping with hurting, and I wanted to try and help, make sure her baby and Blake, her husband, had everything they needed.

Blake was living up in Savannah with his mom, Brandy, so we just started a whole collection and it was so heartening to see how many people came forward. Women offered twenty ounces, a hundred, whatever they had that they could give, and the baby made it a year with all donated milk. I had already been involved with [the] birthing and breastfeeding community, but really this is how I got into the sharing part. This is really when my crusade began.

As with McKenna, donors wanted to know where their milk was going. Many, like Rainey, resisted the alienation that could, would, happen when milk went to an unknown baby through a bank or for-profit company. She had moved from upstate New York to the area with her husband; Robert had a job as a caretaker at a large country estate near Hilton Head. Their family lived in a medium-sized house on the estate. Rainey was a stay-at-home mother to four children, who had the run of the farm, especially while the owners were away, which according to Rainey was most of the time. She was heavily involved in local Christian church activities and a homeschooling group. She prizes education, reading, spending time outside, and being involved in her community. Her children, who ranged in age from one to eight, were well mannered, poised, and healthy.

They always called me "Miss Susan" (for those readers who are not from the South, some young children here are taught to respectfully refer to adults with "Miss" and "Mister" and the adult's first name) and ran out to meet me at my car, asking if they could help bring in anything, telling me about their latest exploits and discoveries, and asking about the baby. She had breastfed each of them for two years. She shared much in common with others I would meet over the next years.

When I met her, she was breastfeeding her youngest child, then just over a year old, but she made about ten ounces a day for us: "I am just one of those lucky women who produce an overabundance [of breast milk] and don't want to see it go down the drain." With her third child she had contacted a milk bank and went through the signing up and testing process so she could donate the overage, but she experienced problems.

She was concerned when she learned what the bank planned to do with her milk. In her discussions with the bank she had discovered that they planned to use two-thirds of the milk for research, while only one-third went to Africa. And while she was thrilled that some was going to Africa (to feed to babies diagnosed with HIV, she assumed), she did not like that it was mostly being used for research, especially since she was not privy to what the research projects were or what they were being used for. "And I already know that milk is good for babies!" she explained. She wanted to have more control over how it was being used; she decided to look for a family with a baby who would consume all of the milk.

I spent many mornings driving to Rainey's in South Carolina with my son. I always took him, not only so he could have a pleasant outing and play with her children but also because there was, I must admit, a performative side: I wanted Rainey to see that he was thriving, partly, I was sure, due to the donated milk he was consuming. I wanted her to know that her milk was being put to good use. Over time, visits became more relaxed, longer, and more sociable. As a new mother, I was happy to ask for, and receive, advice from someone with experience. She helped me understand not just how to defrost and best preserve milk—the basics—but also what to do when the baby had a high fever, how to make and freeze baby food, and how to use breast milk in ways that I would not have imagined.

The morning I picked up the first donation, we hugged, and she told me how thankful and blessed she was to be able to give milk to us. She impressed upon me how important she felt it was to give children breast milk, and she said she admired how hard I was working to ensure a good start for our baby. I was happy to hear this, but I very surprised at how thankful *she* was to be doing this. Meanwhile I had been frankly wondering to myself how I was going to be able to thank her! Several months later she became pregnant with her fifth child. She stopped donating but did make it a personal mission to find a replacement. At the time of writing we remain in touch and she is awaiting baby number six.

Others helped make breast milk sharing possible by setting up or serving as administrators on social media sites, being active in LLL, and making matches. For example, the Facebook page Milky Mommas, founded in 2011 by Christine, is a forum for all things breast milk and beyond. "How did you get into this?" I asked her. "Have you ever been a donor yourself?" She replied,

> I have donated milk personally a few times. I have wet-nursed while babysitting twice, and I pumped within my first week postpartum, after my second baby, to donate to another newborn born the same week who was diagnosed FTT [failure to thrive] when his mom struggled with breastfeeding. We were connected through our IBCLC [international board certified lactation consultant]. I am about to make a donation to a mom for whom I served as birth doula. She struggled with fertility before conceiving the baby, whose birth I attended, and then became pregnant again by total surprise at only four months postpartum! Her milk dried up, but her goal was still to give her daughter breastmilk until at least a year.

Christine then explained that she was a matchmaker for donation relationships: "In addition to my personal donations, I've helped to facilitate informal milk donations during emergency situations for babies who lost their mothers, or whose mothers were incapacitated. For example there we had a situation where a six-week-old breastfed infant mother returned to work, and on her first day back, collapsed unexpectedly, and passed away; I believe [our group] sent over five hundred ounces to the father in the Augusta area."

Another time a mother experienced sepsis after a uterine infection, and her baby had to be kept away from her for two weeks while she was hospitalized and heavily medicated. Her baby "did not do well on formula," so Christine collected and shipped three hundred ounces of milk to northern Michigan, where the family had gone to recover.

I was already familiar with Christine's third example because I knew other people, including McKenna (above), who had donated milk to them. I had been told several versions of the story about a mother who had gone into cardiac arrest when she was pulled over for a traffic violation (all basically in agreement, but differing in a Rashomanlike way, as we might expect, in details), but in Christine's words, "The EMTs were not able to intubate her in a timely manner. She was removed from life support a few days later. Her exclusively breastfed three-month-old son became the recipient of many milk donations over the following months. I helped with finding donors, receiving shipped milk, arranging logistics for milk to be transported from throughout this state and others, and also with storing it until it could be passed on to the father." This story is a remarkable in many ways: when her death was announced on the local parenting boards, many people—friends and strangers—stepped in to help the grieving father with food, child care, supplies, and breast milk, and it shows how this group did far more than simply move milk.

Christine is what my family calls a "nexus person." She knows lots of people in various social groups and is able to bring them together, so it is not surprising that she founded a Facebook group. She explained to me that she wanted it to "provide information and support for women who are or are interested in breastfeeding or breast milk feeding. We have around 2,500 members currently, and a lot of milk-sharing arrangements originated within the group. Like right now, I am assisting a mother who travels between Savannah and Charleston, who has a baby around eight months old. Her baby is going to a gastrointestinal specialist up there because he cannot tolerate formula. He has had many health issues since cessation of breastfeeding. He needs breast milk!"

With women moving away from their own natal families and having children later in life, there is less support for them when they are learning to breastfeed. The rise in occupations such as doula and lactation consultant testify to this. And at times new moms may feel isolated. Christine told me,

I started Milky Mommas because my daughter was almost five months old and the only knowledgeable breastfeeding support I had was my IBCLC and my mom, who breastfed her three children a quarter of a century plus ago. I wanted to get a few women I knew in the same place to talk, to share our experience, and support each other. I thought if I could get a dozen women on the site, then it would be a success. But, there must have been a lot more like me, because everyone kept adding more women who added more women. At one point, we had thousands, and then restructured it to make it more manageable, deleting a significant portion. Then the site began to grow again. Now I have a team to help me run things! So there are really a lot of people out there involved. And you know, I didn't personally know the mom who passed away, I was introduced to her story through a mutual friend on the site. I helped get the donations, and the mutual friend took them back to the family. It is very heartwarming and fulfilling to be part of such an amazing act of love and giving. It makes me so proud of our village of women and the community impact we can have.

Some women became donors after having been donees themselves. Jaye, who was herself an IBCLC, was breastfeeding her son Nero, who was born with a tongue-tie:

I finally got an EMT to [clip the tie] when he was about nine days old, but up to that point I had been hand expressing into his mouth because he just could not suck, and so at about six days or so I developed mastitis [a painful inflammation of the breasts], and my nipples were torn up, and I got an infection so I started pumping because I knew that hand expressing was not going to allow me to make enough milk and it had become clear that my supply was already going down, probably because not enough milk was being removed, or maybe stress was causing my supply to decrease. Anyway, I stared pumping around the clock and I also reached out and was able to augment with donor milk. All in all I had five donors. One was my sister in

Charleston. Then some acquaintances around here (in Atlanta), and then I got some from a local OB (my friend that made the connection). She went and picked up the milk and brought it to my house—I never actually met the mom.

So, I was pumping, breastfeeding, and using donor milk. I was using donated and pumped milk using an SNS. We had OT [occupational therapy] after the tongue-tie but we were using a bottle because he still was not sucking strongly enough. At three months post-OT, he stopped needing extra milk and my supply increased as we finally got it figured out.

But then I had leftover milk, and I was so grateful and I wanted to say "thank you" and I wanted to pay it forward. So when he was eight months old, I reached out on Facebook and I found a mom in need, we met, and I told her that I had a freezer full and I gave it to her. She had a breast reduction before her kids and found that she really could not make enough—she almost could—but she was going to use donor milk as a supplement. I became a regular donor, and I also got another mom to donate to them weekly. We got ten to twenty ounces each to her each week, so between twenty to forty ounces a week, to her for several months. It was really cool to see the baby growing and doing well and I liked the mom a lot. So it was all just coming around full circle. I have a few bags in my freezer but my supply is dwindling, so I am waiting on Facebook to see if anyone has a need.

Pumping and giving are understood as a form of affective labor, of power, and of gratifying altruism, so there are strong emotional ties that bind donors with donees.

Agency

But what about agency within the counternetwork? To what extent is breast milk sharing a self-conscious effort? The degree of agency has implications for the possibility of progressive social action, for notions of responsibility, and for consciousness. Christine's and McKenna's stories certainly suggest that sharing is part of a broader strategy for being part of a community. My own understanding of agency has always included some element of intentionality (see Gell 1998, 16). Many donors plainly stated that they are promoting breastfeeding and breast milk by actively transgressing mandates against sharing issued by institutionalized medicine: they are unruly, cyborgian, lactivist.

The question of agency is important because, among other things, it is future oriented. Now that venture capitalists have entered into the milk race and scientists are working to replicate milk in a lab, the pressure against the sharing counternetwork is bound to increase.

Unequally distributed capital and power shapes how people share milks, filtering who is in or out. Describing his donor pool, Brian mentioned having at least ten different donors, some of whom were regular, long-term donors and others who just gave a few ounces. His explanation was reminiscent of my own experience: "The donors were of a Republican persuasion. They were all stay at home moms and most of them seemed to be doing well [financially]. The doctor was doing very well, the tree farmer seemed to be doing fine, and my colleague's wife [who became a donor], well, I happen to know he comes from a family of means, but they are Christian proselytizers, and they live modestly but are pretty conservative. I mean, my colleague is a huge Rick Santorum supporter so that kind of tells you about his politics."

This profile of his donors surprised Brian and caused him to "recalibrate" some of his ideas:

> Where were the liberals I expected to see? To me, there are two things here, one is my own surprise, which reflects a certain bias on my part, and two, is that the inclination of donors comes from their world view, so what does it say, that here are all these conservatives donating? Is it personal action and philanthropy? I suspect it is deeper than that, something about an idea about the world. But I don't know. One thing I learned from this is that there is a community built up around a need and facilitated by the Internet with people from all political stripes that want to help other people.

When I asked April to describe her donors, she related a similar experience. Their first and most prolific donor, Ashlee, was a military wife living at Fort Stewart, a huge military installation only about forty miles west of her home. She recalled meeting Ashlee for the first time. They had agreed to meet at the local mall, somewhere April said she would not normally go: "We were both a bit wary, or nervous, and we both came with our families. We met at an indoor playground with the kids and it was very friendly. But it was funny too, especially when we learned that she assumed we would not be Caucasian. She did not say this, but I think she thought our names were odd."

April said of her donors, "They were married. And I'd say they were mostly Republicans, but at least one was not. Several were very religious, and by that, I mean Christian. And we had two military families. Racially, most, but not all, were white. I believe one was Hispanic. But interestingly, at the midwife clinic where I had Stella, I noticed that a lot of the patients were military, Republican, white, and rural. Our donors had similar characteristics."

Her next family owned a small farm in rural Georgia, an hour or so away. They also shared with "a lawyer who shipped often from North Carolina, and aside from those three keeping up our supply at the beginning, we had quite a few one-time or small-quantity donors. Two we met on the highway for the exchange (one of those gave us the mother lode!) and we also got some from a doctor in Charleston, and a local photographer. The photographer ended up taking our baby photos of Stella. And then there was another lawyer, and a few others. I'd guess we had at least twelve or fifteen different donors over the two years that we were involved."

When I raised the issue of rejecting donors with April, she explained that she "did not follow-up on a couple of people on the online milk sharing board, but it was usually because I wanted to pass on an offer if someone else was in greater need, for example, if they had a younger baby or if their baby was allergic to formula. Occasionally I passed on a donor because the quantity was too small to warrant shipping costs (which we always paid for)."

When we were looking for donors, several didn't work out. We had at least one donor who wanted us to buy an electric double breast pump for her in exchange for milk and one who called us near the end of our experience with an offer to sell us her supply; we chose not to participate in these opportunities. I was concerned about the incentive for adulteration that commodification might present, and I did not have the money to buy a double pump based on a promise of future milk.

This decision was partly made because we had talked with women who wanted to become donors and expected to build up a stash for us but found that they were, in the end, unable to do it.

The smell, color, texture, and flavor of everyone's milk was slightly different, and although my children seemed to prefer some donor milk to others (and we jokingly called Stephanie's very blue milk "top shelf"), we never encountered a lipase problem or milk rejection situation. But April did: "Stella rejected milk from one donor—the pediatrician from Charleston. We kept it and mixed with other milk as a backup, and eventually used most of it. But [the donor] really was put out by our needing medical records and additional tests. She gave us a copy of her pregnancy test results, but was unwilling to do more. I guess she thought it was overkill." And, as a donor, she was in a position to choose what to give and what to keep. The same can be true for donees.

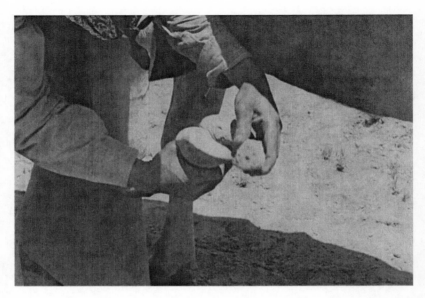

17. Still from the film *Go West* (1925). Friendless, played by Buster Keaton, travels west to make his fortune. Once there, he tries his hand at bronco busting, cattle wrangling, and dairy farming, eventually forming a bond with a cow named Brown Eyes.

Hui

The Maori filmmaker Barry Barclay (1990) argues for filmmaking as *hui*, the term for a gathering or meeting; film assembles people in all stages of production, from preproduction consultation to audience reception. A community coalesces around the film.

Lesley Stern (forthcoming) describes how objects in films animate relationships: in Buster Keaton's 1925 film *Go West*, a stone lodged in a cow's hoof activates a relationship with Friendless, the cowboy.

Objects shape how life happens. We intend ourselves into the world through objects: diamonds, shoes, demolition derby cars, and bags of frozen milk. We embrace, push away, engulf, make, know, or nudge each other through them. Our very identities depend upon our engagement with objects—creation, production, circulation, consumption, divestment, or even rejection. Without them we do not exist. We are transitive in this sense.

Katherine Carroll (2015b) has found that NICU mothers may worry that donor milk will interfere with mother-infant bonding, challenge their new and thus fragile sense of motherhood, or lead their children to reject their breast and the milk it provides. The power of others' milk is threatening. Avoid! Sharers, on the other hand, tend to celebrate milk's power to assemble.

Hoping the baby wouldn't wake up, she read a few pages of Stewart's *Ordinary Affects* (2008) while waiting for the Other Mother to arrive. Witch's water pooled in the gas station parking lot adjacent to a busy strip mall. A familiar souped-up Hummer pulled up. "Hi, I have 'em in the back!" They got out, gave each other a hug, then chatted as they scooped baggies of milk out of one cooler and into another. When they were done, she placed cardboard and a hunk of dry ice on top of the baggies. She often thought of the Other Mother, especially later when she defrosted the bags for her son. Milk = *hui*.

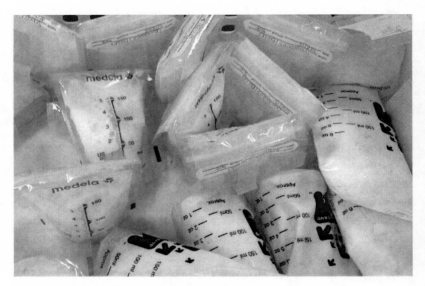

18. Milk, frozen rock hard. Photo by author.

3   Breast Milk Is Best

Charlotte gave birth to a baby girl, but when the nurse first brought the baby to her to nurse, it did not go well. "It is not as easy as you would think," she told me. "And I had a feeding nurse and everything."

Despite the idea that babies and their mothers "just naturally" know how to breastfeed, Charlotte said, "at least in my experience, they don't!" She tried. She tried hard. And Charlotte, who has a PhD in art history from an elite academic institution and is the executive director of a respected regional cultural center, is a woman of no small force. Despite her best efforts, she was unable to produce enough milk for her Ava. She supplemented with formula, she told me, much to the raised brow of her "more bohemian friends who made me feel like I wasn't trying hard enough, like I was not being a good mom."

Because of her experience having friends react to supplementing with formula as tantamount to a kind of moral failure, when I explained that I was writing about my own experience, Charlotte had many questions: Why didn't you use formula? How did you find people? Were they people you already knew, like a relative? How much did you pay them? Was it like a wet nurse? What were the women like? Do you really think it is better than formula? Charlotte had no idea that such a thing was possible.

This chapter presents stories of women and men whose children are donees. Paying attention to the circumstances that enable or discourage sharing shows how it shapes and is shaped by participants. Donors highlight how sharing entails and is entailed by cultural configurations, technological innovations, and the management of risk, all of which underpin the sharing within which identities are enacted. Donors also become entwined in donees' stories and subjectivities, themselves shaped by circulation, technology, and risk.

Since milk sharing has no formal structure, central authority, or insti-tutional rules, participants can change roles over time. Sometimes donors become donees, or donees become donors, or doulas or lactation con-sultants take on the role of either when they give birth themselves. But in the end, reminiscent of the mother::child dyad, donors and donees are in a sense co-constitutive. It is important to keep in mind, however, that the playing field is far from even. The "network" metaphor connotes horizontality, but there are important differences in participants' abil-ity to "hook in" and to shape how milk sharing works. Filters based on class, health, maternal status, and so forth shape, if not determine, who participates and in what capacity. But the organization and power struc-ture of the community are quite flexible. Because participants have the potential to take on various roles, the counternetwork can be described as a heterarchy.

The term "heterarchy" was introduced in the mid-1940s by Warren McCulloch (1945), a neurophysiologist and early cybernetician (influ-enced by Peirce's work in developing a triadic logic). Decades later the term was taken up in anthropology by archaeologists such as Carole Crumley (1995).[1] According to Crumley and Marquardt (1987, 158), "Hierarchies (as opposed to other kinds of structured relations) are composed of an array of elements which are subordinate to others and may be ranked." We are so accustomed to thinking about hierarchy as an ordering principle (in language, logic, and sociopolitical life) that "hierarchy" now acts not as one possible mode of ordering but as a per-vasive structural metaphor and a definition for order itself. In fact, "when hierarchy and order are considered interchangeable, the popular under-standing of chaos—the word of Greek origin for confusion or lack of pattern or plan—opposes hierarchy" (Crumley 1995, 2). But this oppo-sition is false; many structures, from neural networks to cities, can be perfectly orderly while not organized hierarchically. It is worth quoting Crumley (1995, 1–3) here at length:

> This conflation of hierarchy with order makes it difficult to imagine, much less recognize and study, patterns of relations that are complex but not hierarchical. . . . Heterarchy was first employed in a modern context by McCulloch (1945). He examined alternative cognitive struc-

ture(s), the collective organization of which he termed heterarchy. He demonstrated that the human brain, while reasonably orderly, was not organized hierarchically. This understanding revolutionized the neural study of the brain and solved major problems in the fields of artificial intelligence and computer design. To date, it has had little impact on the study of society. . . . Heterarchy may be defined as the relation of elements to one another *when they are unranked or when they possess the potential for being ranked in a number of different ways.* . . . While hierarchy undoubtedly characterizes power relations in some societies, *it is equally true that coalitions, federations, and other examples of shared or counterpoised power abound.* The addition of the term heterarchy to the vocabulary of power relations reminds us that *forms of order exist that are not exclusively hierarchical and that interactive elements in complex systems need not be permanently ranked relative to one another.* In fact, it may be in attempts to maintain a permanent ranking that flexibility and adaptive fitness is lost. . . . Hierarchical relationships among elements at one spatial scale or in one dimension (members of the same club) may be hierarchical at another (the privilege of seniority in decision making). [emphasis added]

In this framework elements shift and change according to context; decisions are made on the basis of superlocal considerations and power is relational. I am especially intrigued by milk sharing as a highly flexible and adaptive heterarchical counternetwork not only insofar as it is highly efficient (once our family started making connections, not one day went by when we were unable to provide our children with donated milk, and we continued to receive offers after we had stopped pursuing donations) but also in that it shows us, especially as milk sharing becomes more well known and overtly contested by powerful institutions, how "atomized, mundane acts can shift into the realm of contentious politics" (Bayat 2010).

Breast Milk Is Best

"A diamond is forever" is one of the most successful advertising taglines ever written; almost all American adults are familiar with it, the major-

ity of American women own at least one diamond, and most engagements are accompanied by the purchase of a diamond (Falls 2014).
Another is Nike's "Just Do It!" Like these commercial examples, the
phrase "breast milk is best" has had tremendous success. I heard count-
less people use these exact words to describe why they gave or sought
milk. Contributing to the construction of breast milk as type, "breast
milk is best" is tantamount to "white gold."

We know by looking at the phenomenal rise in breastfeeding rates since
the 1970s that institutional efforts to increase breastfeeding have worked,
creating a strong imperative to provide babies with breast milk. In fact
some women, like Charlotte, report that as a result of the cultural pressure
to breastfeed *no matter what*, they have been made to feel guilty or as if
they were somehow lesser parents as a result of doing anything else.

Dr. Martin, a local neonatologist, expressed concerns about the mandate placed on moms to breastfeed as she reflected upon an open secret
in her NICU: "With the 'breast milk is best,' maybe there is a point of too
much pressure. When is too much? I ask myself that sometimes because
I have seen NICU moms—who are told to go home and pump—bring in
formula and say that it is milk, or bring in a ton of breast milk when just
the day before they had not been able to pump or anything, and I know
[the milk they bring] is from a sister or friend, and we just go with it."

Feelings of both guilt and gratitude loom large. Some moms felt that
their devotion, love, or desire to be a good parent *was* challenged when
they couldn't exclusively breastfeed. As donor Claire recognized, on
behalf of her donee, "It is just very difficult for those who cannot generate their own supply." Or, as recipient Kristina put it,

My firstborn was premature and he was also on Nutramigen [a formula that markets itself as "a hypoallergenic formula proven to manage colic due to cow's milk protein allergy"], which he projectile
vomited across the room. And it was really bad. My second one, I
breastfed for over a year with no problems, and the same with my
third. My fourth was in NICU for eight days because he was premature, and I was going up there to the hospital and doing my best to
breastfeed him, but when you are not with the baby it is hard to keep
up, and it was just not happening, so after that . . . we used formula,

which I hated to do, but it was alright. And then this one, my fifth, was fine at first, but then we started having issues. Except this time I went to donor milk. These moms are so awesome, and I just have had a great experience. Some people ask about disease or dangers but they [the donors] are not out [to get] anything, they just do it for the babies. All I provide is the bags, and I talked to some of them about this; I wish I could do more. Because this just means the world to us.

When I asked her what her husband thought about sharing, she said, "At first, he thought it sounded crazy! 'You are gonna go get milk from some other lady?' But, when he saw that the baby was feeling so much better, he was like 'Here is some gas money! Go get what you need.'" Kristina explained to others in her breastfeeding group that "their idea that sharing milk is weird is just because of our day and time: what is weird about it? We are just not used to thinking about it like this. Hey, they all drink cow's milk! But then I think, well, just look at me! I never even knew [sharing] was an option. And I have five kids! Sure, I knew all about the banks, and I did look into that when my first was having such a rough time [with formula]. I called around and did research, but what I discovered was that it was very expensive, if you can even get it. And there was no way we could pay that. But in all my searching for the right bank, I never saw anything about sharing for free. But that was in 2006, so I think that more people are into it now, but back then, it just wasn't available. Now that I know it's an option, I hope more people do it."

Kristina is inspired by the altruism and affective labor she attributes to her donors. She believes "they would not do it [donate] if they were having problems," meaning that if donors had health issues that would create problems for babies, they would not participate. She is hoping to develop a frozen supply so she can donate:

I am taking Reglan, to up my supply, and I am almost to where I am caught up with him. But gosh, I would love to help someone else. I want to find a baby I can donate to regularly, like our regular donor does for us. I live near a lot of people who are interested in doing this, but it's not easy. Like I have this one girl that lives just down the road, and she gave me some in the beginning, but then she had to go out of town and it was just too much for her to keep up the amount by pumping while she was on the road, so she called me and explained that she might not be able to provide us with forty or fifty ounces a week like she wanted to. But it seems like there are more people who need it than there are people who want to donate. There really is a lot of need. I check all the local sites on Facebook, all the ones near me, in Georgia or even Florida or Alabama, but I mean I have five kids so it is hard for me to go too far. Then again, I will do what I have to do. I don't want to see him suffering.

Many women described variations on affective states such as care and love, gratitude, and the desire to help, as well as the relationships between demand and supply and the pressure to conform to the breast-milk-is-best dictum. As April recounted,

When I tell people about milk sharing, they are like, "Oh my God! I threw so much away! I wish I would have known—I would have given it to someone!" Anyway, I found it really confusing to know whether breast milk really is better from the literature available, so I just went with what I thought was the right thing. They need to study these donation babies. I wanted the breastfeeding connection, but then again, is it the milk or is it the action? How long is long enough? But gosh, it was painful. Cracked nipples, blood, pumping! But later, it became really pleasant. And the imperative! They make you feel like you are not doing right by the baby if you do not breast feed, even though God knows I tried. I found that La Leche League does not really make allowances for people who are more moderate. I find them too militant. The group here made me feel like I didn't try hard enough, but then they do not have experience with breast surgery. I don't think they really know enough to say. I tried to read the books and all but I never read anything about donation.

Like April, mothers who can produce only a low supply, are not able to pump at work, or are suffering from genetic or medical conditions preventing them from producing any or enough milk may also chase donated milk. Caretakers of a baby whose mother has died, or fathers who cannot produce milk, grandparents who find themselves caring for a baby, adoptive or foster parents, and others may all want to feed their baby breast milk. And given the imposing push for milk against formula by pretty much every authoritative institution out there, who can blame them?

Leah described an experience similar to others I heard: "My daughter is two now, and even though I had a low supply from the beginning, we have continued to nurse throughout with the help of donor milk. So, we had to use an SNS for the bulk of the time." While many mothers stop breastfeeding at the milestone age of one, feeling like they have "made it," others like Leah continue nursing until age two and even beyond. In my own experience our first adopted child was allergic to cow's milk, so we kept using donated milk until he was about eighteen months old and was able to tolerate goat's milk.

Our second baby was able to drink cow's milk (and consume other milk products, like yogurt), and although we stopped actively seeking donated milk when she reached the milestone age of one, we continued to provide her with the milk we still had combined with cow's milk until we ran out, around the time she turned a year and a half. These milestone ages were turning points for others as well. April said she was

> starting to feel guilty [asking for donated milk] because Rory was getting older, so I was no longer vying to be the first in line. My goal had been a year but at nine months she was eating food and so I didn't feel right taking it. But then we were on the last layer in the fridge, but someone contacted me and said she had a two-month supply and would we take it? Rory was taking about twenty-four ounces a day, and this was still a lot, and this woman was pumping at work and had an oversupply and was looking for someone to use it because her donee had fallen through and she was on the way to Florida. She was emptying her freezer anyway and said, "I will be in Savannah at five o clock, I have my records and can be at exit so and so," and so, in this case, she actually found us.

This was somewhat unusual, but in April's own mind, although Rory's need had decreased, the milk might be wasted if they did not receive it. She sent her husband to the exit to pick it up.

The fact that our daughter was able to easily transition from donor milk to cow's milk was part of our decision to stop seeking milk, but we recognized families with infants in our network who might need the milk more than we did. For example, I knew from Facebook that Amanda's daughter Marjorie has cystic fibrosis, a genetic disorder that causes her body to produce an excess of thick, sticky mucus. When I talked with her, Amanda explained that the disease primarily affects her daughter's lungs and pancreas, with her pancreas being severely insufficient. Marjorie has to take pancreatic enzymes with every feeding so her body can properly digest and absorb her food. Her body requires extra calories to make up for nutrients lost to inefficient digestion and to compensate for the extra effort her body needs to digest food and to breathe. Amanda explained,

> Factoring in the need for extra food plus just the amount of stress created in just caring for her cystic fibrosis, I wasn't producing enough of my own milk. She was consistently under the 3% line for weight. We were pushed, hard, to use human milk fortifier (which is quite pricey) and to supplement with formula. I had nursed my first daughter for a year and with Marjorie I wanted to go even further. I loved the nursing bond and providing antibodies for my special needs daughter who requires all the protection and help she can get. But it was difficult. By four months, I was having to pump most of her feedings. At six months, I wasn't producing enough milk on my own and began supplementing with formula, which I hated to have to do. Two friends knew of our struggles and how stressful things were for us. They stepped forward and began bringing me bags of their precious milk. We have had many friends and family offer various kinds of help throughout our journey with our daughter's cystic fibrosis, but this was truly a unique way to help our little girl. I was nervous to reach out further to strangers, but I joined HM4HB on Facebook and a local mom donated almost forty ounces to me. Hopefully one day we'll have another child and I can bless another family with my milk. It's an overwhelming feeling of love and support, and I'd like to extend it to others.

Amanda's comments demonstrate that milk sharing is a form of affective labor, which colors the emotional experience of participation in what Carroll has called "care work" (Carroll 2015a).

A Deserving Baby

Because we were constantly studying the local milk-sharing websites, we came to know other families like Amanda's, if only vicariously. In 2010 our quest for donated milk was thwarted on multiple occasions by Jennifer and Robert, who needed milk for their son, baby Joah. Jennifer, we came to know, had a low supply due to breast-reduction surgery, but she was impressively active in finding donated milk for her baby. We thought we were being pretty vigilant and had a good system for checking the boards, but she was even better! She frequently replied more quickly than anyone else to postings that offered of a good-sized stash, and we quickly realized that she was willing to drive anywhere, much farther than we could reasonably do (and we had more or less decided that we, or actually my husband, would drive up to four hours for a large supply and even farther for a very large load, while I would take the children with me on shorter runs). At one point Jennifer even held a party for local donors, which we thought was a wonderful strategy for meeting and thanking all of the counternetwork moms but also for ensuring Joah had a steady supply.

When we had our second child in 2012, we were astonished to see that Jennifer and now baby Leona were back in what we joked was a competition. It really felt like that at times. April had also used this language when she described her last donor, who "was so excited to find someone who could use her milk. She had so much, and had taken so much care, labeling everything and freezing it just right, and really it seemed like she found us! But at the beginning you have to work hard, and search, and we felt like we had to compete to get it, but it always worked out. I mean in the beginning, we were so vigilant." Like April, we never actually ran out, though we came close a few times. Other donees reported a similar dynamic of hustling to ensure a solid supply, worrying when the freezer was getting empty, but then always, or almost always, finding a donor before running out.

Finding donors or making what some participants call a "milky match" required constantly checking Facebook and MilkShare. Some donors had very specific ideas about who would get their milk, which is part of the reason that parents seeking donor milk often revealed why they needed it, describing their own medical or social conditions or their babies' allergies, illnesses, or diseases. Posted donee narratives take on a somewhat regular character: mothers looking for breast milk strive through these narratives to appear, well, motherly, appreciative, and truly needy. Missy's request is not atypical: "Hi! I have twin ten-month olds who I have been giving donated milk to almost exclusively through the generosity of HM4HB mothers! I can't breastfeed because I am being treated for cancer myself. We will be in [the area] visiting relatives and would greatly, greatly appreciate any donations to see us through our time in [the area]! We can meet or drive for donations! Thank you!"

Melody also expressed a need for breast milk, a need that, if unmet, would force the use of formula: "Hello there! I am a mother of a beautiful baby girl named Elly who is six months of age. We live in [small town]. My supply has basically dried up. We depend on donor milk to help feed my sweet girl that precious breast milk. I supplement with formula when necessary. Any sized donations in a 150-mile radius would be greatly appreciated!! I can replace bags. Please PM me or tag me in this post if you can help!" In our own posts, we usually stated that our adopted children were using donated milk; at least two of our donors were themselves adopted and had looked specifically for adoptees to donate to.

Other donees mentioned problems pumping at work when they made a public request for help. This is a class concern; working women across the board may have little time or privacy at work, although those with higher-status jobs tend to have more say in their working conditions and thus are better positioned to pump at work.

For some parents a minor breastfeeding issue that still allowed them to feed might be exacerbated by having to pump at work. Kaya, for example, was able to easily breastfeed Jolene, her first child, but when she had her second baby two years later, even though she had experienced a really healthy pregnancy, she was unable to breastfeed: "Parker came out really fast and had some jaw issues, so she just had trouble latching on. I ended up pumping and giving her a bottle, and that went fine, but then she was unwilling to go to the breast after that. So, when I had to go back to work, part time, I just wasn't able to keep up." Donor milk makes up the difference created by the resulting (and frustrating) loss of supply.

Kaya, a well-educated and savvy archivist at a research center, reads the link between women's bodies and political economy pretty plainly: "The breast milk issue is policy related. All of the major health institutions, the AMA [American Medical Association], WHO, and so on, are all recommending breast milk, but American labor policy just does not support it. Most women have to go back to work after they run through what little maternity leave they have. And once that happens, it is very difficult to continue breastfeeding."

Some parents, like Kaya, are prevented from breastfeeding due to the requirements of their employment. Brianna, one of our regular donors, for example, was deployed to Iraq while her child was still at the breast. The last time I picked up a donation from Brianna she asked me if I could help her find a donor for her young daughter. Here was a woman who not only had a willingness to breastfeed and a more than sufficient supply of breast milk but was compelled to stop breastfeeding because of her military obligations. I asked if there was not some way that she might extend her maternity leave; Brianna explained that it was possible but that unfortunately her family could not afford it. They were hoping that her husband could be stationed doing drone strikes from a facility in the United States since that specialty paid well. Only then could she afford to return home to care for her young children.

But even mothers who can stay at home might turn to donated milk to supplement a low supply. After having breast surgery Caroline was unable to produce enough milk for her son. She began using formula but then discovered through casual conversations with other mothers after LLL meet-ups that there was a milk-sharing community up and running. Caroline was able to supplement her own supply "without resorting to formula" until Velma was a year old and started drinking cow's milk. Caroline explained that, while she was nervous at first, she found sharing to be "strange but also wonderful." And it was fulfilling an imperative she felt "to provide healthy nourishment to my baby—an imperative that came from doctors but also from random strangers who suggested that of course breastfeeding is the best." She reported that, not unlike being pregnant, which apparently prompted strangers to comment on her body and even touch her belly, having an infant with you invites unsolicited comments about the importance of breastfeeding, which she was doing, but not without some help.

I agreed with her that it just seemed "more natural" to feed a baby breast milk, especially when you read the ingredients on a package of formula, although we suspected that formula would be fine, if necessary. Caroline and I had to laugh together because as formula babies ourselves, we seemed to have turned out all right. We also had to laugh about the quality of "formula poo," which as any new parent can tell you becomes a major topic of observation and conversation. Formula poo is drier, thicker, and pasty (or pebbly), brownish, and, well, malodorous, whereas breast milk poo is mushy, yellow, and lightly fragranced (with a sweeter note). This difference is partly the result of different proteins in each: formula contains more casein, which takes longer to digest and thus is denser and smellier. Whey-heavy breast milk slides through the digestive system more easily, with concomitant results. The scientific community might view our conclusions as folk wisdom, but we read this poo oracle as a sign that we were doing the right thing, that breast milk is indeed superior to formula.

And besides, Velma was healthy and happy, partly, Caroline believed, due to the high-quality breast milk she was drinking. Caroline pumped and breastfed and had located several regular and some large one-time donors, and she had purchased a big freezer in which to store her supply. She also had some "fly-by donors" who gave her smaller amounts; these women were passing through town and pumping while away from their baby at home. She met a few of these near I-95, the highway that runs along the East Coast from Maine to Miami, to drop a fresh supply that they would not be able to freeze or use. She discovered that donors were sometimes even more thankful to her for taking the milk than she was for receiving it. My experience was not dissimilar.

Others in the network addressed the issue of gratitude. Naomi told me that it is vital that "people who do this appreciate that those who are donating are taking time from their family and lives to be helpful to others. Those who use the milk are so grateful, but it is hard to have to count on others to feed your child. Every time you use donor milk, there is a little bit of sadness that you can't provide for your child, along with the joy and appreciation that there are good people out there doing this for others." But she was also awash in thankfulness:

It meant a lot to us to have donors. I literally cried when we got some of our donations. I was terrified to go through what we went through with our first. We know now that he was in pain constantly from the formula, which caused screaming and no sleep. He would only sleep for half an hour or an hour at a time, day or night until he was two-and-a-half years old. It caused me to have postpartum depression, as I never slept, and just held a crying child a lot of my time. So it was a *really* big deal for us to try and avoid formula, in case she has the same food intolerances/allergies.

Not everyone who shared their feelings experienced the sadness Naomi felt for a perceived failure to meet expectations or the guilt that plagued Charlotte. April found that in swallowing the "breast milk is best" rhetoric and related guilt, she discovered a liberatory moment:

Maybe I should have worked harder, but it worked out. I wanted it to be easy, so if I have another [child], I may see a lactation consultant beforehand. But I was so happy that we could be part of this [sharing community] and, well, am I too bourgie [bourgeois]? I could still have a glass of wine and plus Gerald could help feed Rory. Does that sound wrong? I really wanted to do it! But I tried to appreciate the freedoms I had, and see it as sweet, and find ways to give back to the moms. I would not go back and NOT have the [reduction] surgery now; I was so self-conscious and it was so painful, and I couldn't even run, and that sucked, and I was frustrated, but I have no regrets now.

These comments point to the special relationships that develop among participants. Many donors I met expressed intense thankfulness at not only being able to donate but also at the fact that donees like myself were taking the time and energy to look for milk. There was a lot of warm hugging and mutual support, ongoing photos and updates about weight and health, and so on. In the beginning I wondered if my own stories were unique, but when I started interviewing others I discovered that they were decidedly not.

One father underscored the wonderful sense of adventure I felt in sharing: "I had a great time collecting the milk with Carson. It was fun and had a purpose. I had fun with the people. I enjoyed visiting with them and it was almost like a distant relative relationship. I would drive up to an hour and a half [to pick up milk]. . . . I loved this because it meant that I had an opportunity to bond with Carson. . . . I always took her with me and it was a special time for us to be together, she was little and liked to sleep or ride in the car."

Then again, like relationships with distant relatives can be, contact between donors and donees was fleeting and serendipitous. The relationships created around the technologized exchange of milk were often brief. I found few examples of friendships outlasting the donation schedule, even when feelings were wholehearted and donation persisted over many months. But most women did at the every least report feeling on "common ground as women," "part of a larger community of parents," or "part of a village that was coming through for the children." And, as I explained, most interviewees were white, married in a heterosexual relationship, and middle class. Echoing my own experience with these gratitude-filled relationships, April said,

> Some people were wealthy and others were struggling, but nobody seemed *really* bad off. We had some upper middle-class people, you know, two-car professional families with multiple kids, a big TV, a house, that kind of thing. And military—lot of military! And then the farm people. But, they had nice cars, and Christmas cards where everyone is wearing J. Crew outfits. Probably about half were clearly Republicans and no advanced degree, but we also had a doctor and a lawyer. Actually the group as a whole reminded me a little of the people at the midwife clinic. There were people drawn to natural birth, kind of like yuppies but over thirty with money and a good education, left leaning and liberal who don't want an epidural—I guess I would call this group slightly bohemian. And then there were the hippy [*sic*], incense people that wore wraparounds and asked a lot questions about eating placentas. And then there were the really young ones, with little education, who were stay at home, back-to-basics moms, and it seemed like they were very Republican. They were usually white, but not hillbilly, and not urban yuppies either. The milk donation thing followed along these lines. But I *never* dis-

cussed politics, because we are quite liberal, and we really only talked about milk, how the babies were developing, how cute Rory was, that kind of thing. The other moms liked to hold Rory—Amy especially, and Rory liked her—and she sent us notes telling us how honored she was to give her milk to a deserving baby. They were as excited and felt as good about this as I did!

But what about the donees? Like the donors, they were also primarily white, married, and middle class but were decidedly less Christian, with a tendency toward higher education and left-leaning politics. Carolina, Kaya, Naomi, April, Miranda, and I, for example, all work, have college or postgraduate degrees of some kind, are married to white-collar professionals who also have college or postgraduate degrees, and are overtly liberal in our political and cultural views. We also all have the time, money, know-how, and energy to do research on donor milk and on formula and to pursue donors using Internet technology.

Some donors, like Myra, only gave once, gifting their entire overage to one person, in this case our daughter. "My son never really took to a bottle when I went back to work," she explained. "He just he waits for my lunch break! So I had a freezer stash that needed a home. It makes me so happy to know that your daughter has thrived on my donor milk!" Donees, on the other hand, may assume the role of milk recipient for a year or more, so their activity "becomes more professionalized," as my husband described it, once donees learn the ropes and get a routine. One of the benefits of knowing the "secrets of the trade" is that families can move around the country, even the world, and be able to access milk because the underlying infrastructure has been replicated in locations all across the United States and indeed around the world.

For example, when we traveled to visit grandparents, we easily used the HM4MB and MilkShare sites to locate donors in California and Arizona. Women not only provided an ample supply for us while we were there but gave us enough extra to save in a freezer for future trips to the West Coast. Interestingly these donors did not conform to the donor profile I had come to recognize in my own regional counternetwork. Our donors out West, for example, worked, were not overtly Christian, and were highly educated. We also did not engage in the forms of sociality one might expect to see in the South, where any person to-person exchange or business is not necessarily but very likely to be preceded by small talk and storytelling, with milk exchange being no different. Milk sharing brings together people who may never otherwise have a chance to sit down and get to know one another, in an atmosphere of generosity and common ground, and thus can foster new social relationships based on experience rather than stereotype. I suspect and would indeed not be at all surprised if the demographics of the milk-sharing community with its epicenter in Savannah, Georgia, turn out to be somewhat regionally specific.

Then again, even as cultural and political regionalism is real, the composition and the landscape of family forms in the South, as in the United States in general, are undergoing transformation. New religious configurations, the growing acceptance of alternative family forms, and emerging reproductive technologies all have a place in shaping milk sharing in and around Georgia.

In Georgia, with a total population of around 9,687,653 people, 54 percent identify as white and 31 percent identify as African American, while only 9 percent identify as Hispanic (the fastest-growing group). Only 27,057 people are Arab Americans, and of these, half are Egyptian (less than 1 percent of the total population counted in the 2010 census); on a national scale Muslims made up 0.8 percent of the population in 2010 (with 2.6 million people) and are predicted to constitute 1.7 percent by 2030 (largely due to immigration and a higher-than-average fertility rate) (Pew Research Center 2011). And although there are relatively few Muslims living in the South, milk sharing offers them opportunities to continue participating in "milk siblingship" (Altorki 1980; Cole 2010; Parkes 2004, 2005).

Milk sharing can also pose significant concerns for both donors and donees who are Muslim. Just consider the complications that may be posed, for example, if a Muslim family receives donated milk from a milk bank: banks often mix together three separate milks from anonymous donors. Just who and where are their newly minted milk siblings? Participation by Muslim families in national and international milk sharing networks may affect the kinds of relationships being negotiated, as does the shifting panorama of family forms.

Same-sex sexual activity became legal in Georgia only in 1998, and while some cities such as Atlanta maintained a domestic partnership registry for same-sex couples, until the landmark Supreme Court decision of *Obergefell v. Hodges* (Kennedy 2015), Amendment 1 to Georgia's constitution made it illegal for the state to perform or recognize same-sex marriages or civil unions.[2] But many same-sex couples live in Georgia (the gay population constitutes about 3.5 percent of the total population), no state laws prohibit same-sex adoption, and plenty of gay couples in Georgia are raising children.[3] On a national scale the 2010 national census reported 270,000 children living with same-sex couples, 110,000 of whom were adopted (a 100 percent increase over the 2000 census reports but still less than 1 percent of the total child population). Some of these parents are unable to produce breast milk but are subject to the "breast milk is best" messaging and concomitant condemnation of using formula. They may want to give their children donated breast milk.

Drawing on new reproductive technology, some couples, or even singles, use in vitro fertilization, which can result in multiple births (famously difficult to keep up with through breastfeeding, especially when there are more than two infants). Other would-be parents, like Rob and Chance, choose surrogacy, hiring a woman to be implanted with a fertilized egg or eggs (using their own or donated sperm and/or egg) and carry the fetus to term. Gestational surrogacy involves implanting the surrogate with an egg (usually an intended mother's, but the egg could also be a donor egg) that has been fertilized in vitro (usually by an intended father's sperm, but it could be donor sperm), a situation in which the surrogate is not genetically related to the embryo.

With traditional surrogacy a surrogate egg is fertilized (naturally or artificially), so the surrogate is genetically related to the embryo (which results in a more complicated legal situation). Although the practice of surrogacy in the United States remains somewhat problematic because it is highly contested legal terrain, there were more than two thousand surrogate babies born in 2014. There is a wide range of legislation on surrogacy: the state of California has the most permissive laws, New York bans it, and in Washington DC it can even carry criminal penalties. Interestingly many American surrogacy agencies say that most of their clients—gay, straight, married, or single—are international, with foreign couples headed to the United States for surrogate pregnancies (Lewin 2014). The cost of an American surrogacy can be as much as $150,000, and many Americans have opted to pay surrogates abroad in places where it is legal but much less expensive, for example, in India, Russia, Mexico, or Thailand, thus participating in what some scholars call a subset of medical tourism: "fertility tourism" or "reproductive tourism" (Matorras 2005).

And, as Elly Teman (2010) argues in her ethnographic study *Birthing a Mother*, a surrogate mother, what one of my donors called a "surro-mom," performs an elaborate distancing act in order to emotionally detach from the baby while forming close and at times enduring relationships with the intended mother. And indeed Patty, a surrogate mother I interviewed, had continued a relationship with the intended fathers of her "surro-baby" by providing donated milk and was attempting to become pregnant with her intended fathers' second baby.

Patty had become involved with surrogacy after having three of her own children. She was talking to her husband one day about how much she loved being pregnant and breastfeeding, and he had suggested surrogacy. It took her a while to find the right couple, but she had "fallen instantly in step" with Edgar and Roberto. She was very proud of being able to help them create a family by carrying the baby and then providing milk not only for him but for three other donees as well.

There were other surrogates in our network. A recent offer by Jessica on HM4HB Georgia stated that she is three weeks' postpartum as a gestational surrogate to boy/girl twins for "lovely parents in the Midwest." She explains that

> originally, the parents and I discussed I would pump for their babies, pack, and ship the milk to them; however after delivery . . . the family left and the parents have decided not to receive my milk due to the packing and shipping costs of sending frozen milk. So I currently have over 90 ounces of milk frozen in Medela bags. I plan to continue pumping every 3–4hrs until June 3 (I have a 4 week vacation planned end of June thus I would like at least 2 weeks to slowly wean my milk supply before leaving on vacation). At each pumping, with the Medela

Symphony, I average about 3.50z–50z each breast. Is anyone interested in the milk bags I currently have frozen and/or the milk I will be pumping up until June 19? Please FB Message me if you're interested.

What was striking to me was the fact that successful sharing contains a performative aspect here for donors—of parenthood, of altruistic providing, of being competent, of being part of a broader imagined community of mothers, and of trust.

With sites like HM4HB having just celebrated its fifth year in existence at this writing, ideas about the relative good of milk sharing are becoming more common. When I explained in 2010 to my children's doctor and her nurses what we were doing, they were very interested to hear this, but they had never heard of informal milk sharing and did not seem concerned. By 2012, when I asked my doctor and the nurses about it again, they told me that there were still no other families in their office that had discussed milk sharing with them (although there may have been people doing it). April also said that the "lactation consultant at my pediatrician's office was surprised and thought that it was really cool. But, she really only knew about the hospital version."

When Sarah found that she had built up an oversupply as a result of pumping to send milk with her son Whitaker to morning care at a local church, she decided to become a donor. She asked her own lactation consultant about health care issues and what tests she might need to take or to show her donee but found that she "didn't really know anything about it, but then she did some research, and brought me a questionnaire that I filled out for my recipient, who had not asked me for any of that more specific information." Interestingly when the lactation consultant herself had a second child, she also ended up taking advantage of this new practice by using donated milk and then later becoming a donor herself.

One aspect of sharing that my own friends and family did ask me about—a part of this new practice that they "were concerned about" when they learned of our involvement (which usually meant that they really did not think it was a very good idea)—had to do with the issue of trust. How do you know this is not going to make the baby sick? I mean, who is this woman anyway? How do you know her? Why don't you use formula? This giving of advice (use formula, fool!) in the guise of questions reminds me of Wolf's (2013) description of American-style "total motherhood" in which mothers seek to avoid all risks at all costs instead of managing inevitable risks. Given the issues of chemical, bacterial, and heavy-metal contamination, along with the possibilities of disease or even deliberate adulteration of pumped or shared breast milk, as well as the apparent, or even imagined, dangers of formula, donors and donees navigate the risks that are suggested to them by popular discourse. And while donors and donees have different roles, their identities are mutually constructed through not only material exchange but also gratitude, a shared concern with parenting, and a kind of interdependent love: each is necessary for the other to exist. But taking donors and donees as a group we see patterns as well as idiosyncrasies with regard to why people become involved, how they manage risks, and with whom they chose to work.

But actors other than donors and donees help advance milk sharing as a love practice. And as we expect in a social organization characterized by heterarchy, people occupy different roles over time and exert themselves in small and large ways according to circumstances. But how is the heterarchical counternetwork advanced? How does trust come to pervade it? Although activism is diverse and contested, the cumulative effect of individual, mundane acts is to shape the set of norms associated with the sharing infrastructure and to push the (re)production of the counternetwork. (L)activists, who see breast milk as a sacred, quasi-magical liquid that should repel profane commodification, shape this counternetwork in important ways.

The Milky Circle

The Milky Way, our galaxy, as a feature in the night sky, was referred to in classical Latin as *via lacteal* or *circulus lacteus*, a term derived from the Greek *galaxias* (an adjective, as in *galaxias kyklos*), literally "milky circle." In Greek mythology, Athena brought baby Heracles (the love child of Zeus and the mortal Alcmene) to Hera to breastfeed so that he would become immortal. When Hera realized who the baby was, she pushed him away, spraying drops of milk, which then became the Milky Way. You can see these drops turning into stars in *The Origin of the Milky Way*, a Renaissance painting by Tintoretto. In fact the word *galaxy* derives from the Greek word for milk, *γάλα* (gala).

The alchemists' symbol for solar system and galaxy is the same as that used for the sun. In the earliest known accounts of minerals gold was compared to the sun; it was seen as sunlike in its life-giving and universal warmth and color. When we learn that the alchemists' symbol for gold is the same as that as used for the sun, we see the phrase "white gold" deepen. This symbol representing galaxy, sun, and gold—a circle with a dot in the center—also happens to look like a breast. Perhaps activists who promote milk as a community resource, who refer to themselves as "lactivists," might try the more ambitious-sounding "galactivist."

In *The Republic of Therapy* (2010) Vinh-Kim Nguyen uses the term "therapeutic citizenship" to describe how people living with HIV use confession and storytelling to appropriate antiretroviral drugs as a set of rights and responsibilities in a context where disclosure of HIV status can lead to abandonment and shame. In this way therapeutic citizenship is attached to a biomedical condition in which disclosure translates into life-sustaining medical care.

Similarly, galactic citizenship is practiced by sharers narrating need

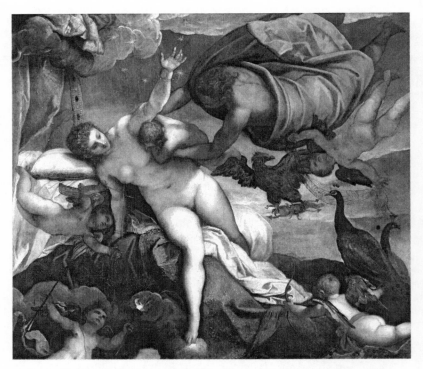

19. Jacopo Tintoretto, *The Origin of the Milky Way*, c. 1575. Oil on canvas. https://commons.wikimedia.org/wiki/File:Jacopo_Tintoretto_-_The_Origin_of_the_Milky_Way_-_Yorck_Project.jpg.

when access to mothers' milk, viewed as necessary to healthy life, is not available. In NICU units banked milk is supplemented with the costly Human Milk–Based Human Milk Fortifier, produced by Prolacta. It is difficult to find up-to-date pricing on fortifier, but Richard Lopez (2013) has reported that a four-ounce bottle of pasteurized human milk cost $56, or $14 an ounce, and that Prolacta estimated the cost of feeding an infant the fortifier ranges from $5,600 to $10,000 per hospital stay. For small babies (who take between 202.8 and 4431.8 milliliters per feeding) in hospitals it is insurance, the state, or the hospital itself that generally subsidizes or covers the costs of providing fortifier, but once a baby is discharged there is no coverage that could even begin to approach the budget required to supply processed human milk to a healthy full-term baby at home for a year.

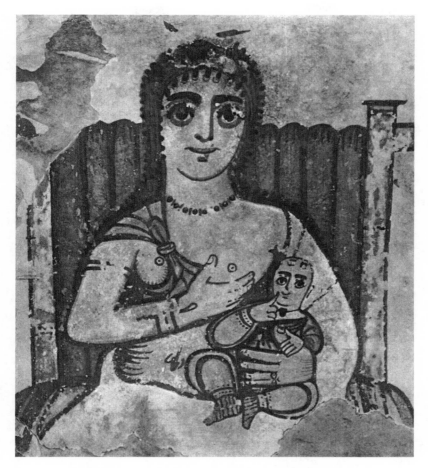

20. Isis nursing infant Harpocrates, third-century wall painting (Karanis, an agricultural town in Greco-Roman Egypt, near Fayum). Note the circle/dot details representing the breast. http://www.umich.edu/~kelseydb/Karanis/KM4.2990_isis.gif.

The demand for milk far outweighs supply. This is the context in which mothers (and fathers) perform, confess, and enact a style of parenting that values breast milk. As with Nguyen's HIV patients, developing the ability to "tell a good story" is key to successfully participating in milk sharing. Donees describe themselves and their babies as needy and deserving while the healthy, lactating mother is cast, like the life-giving sun, as the ultimate universal donor.

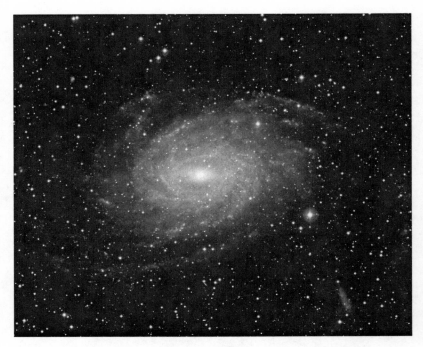

21. Wide Field Imager view of a Milky Way lookalike, NGC6744. Photo from the European Southern Observatory's MPG/ESO 2.2 meter telescope, La Silla, Chile. http://www.eso.org/public/images/eso1118a/.

Less than a century after Tintoretto's rendering of "ga-lactation," Galileo's telescope told us that the Milky Way was made up of individual stars, not a band of light.

Most scientists thought all of the stars in the universe resided in the Milky Way until 1923, when Edwin Hubble discovered a star, dubbed V1, in the outer regions of Andromeda, proving the existence of stars outside of our own galaxy. Astronomers would come to realize that our own galaxy, thought to contain between 100 billion and 400 billion stars and at least 100 billion planets, was just one among billions (Villard 2012a, 2012b). Even more powerful technologies now suggest that our Milky Way looks like NGC6744, a nearby spiral galaxy, *only* about 30 million light years away.[1] Remarkably this galaxy seen from a bird's-eye view resembles the symbol for gold, the sun, and a breast.

4   Lactivism

I recently ran into one of our family's milk donors, Jill, in a newly opened
Whole Foods store in our area. Swaddled against her body, in a Moby
Wrap, was her new little daughter. Jill had regularly donated milk, about
twenty ounces a week, to our first child, and I usually visited her and
her firstborn, a son, in their home just outside of Savannah. Jill's husband is in the military; she is a stay-at-home mom, practices attachment
parenting, is active in a Christian homeschooling group, and is vehe-
mently against childhood vaccines. What really struck the anthropologist
in me was the combination of these values, usually associated with the
political right wing, with her leftist-sounding critiques of profit-driven
business. She promoted sharing in our community by becoming a donor,
advocating donation through word of mouth, and participating in the
local Facebook milk-sharing group. Even though La Leche League does
not officially support milk sharing, Jill had invited me to attend local LLL
meetings to meet additional donors. "I am a lactivist," she had joked.

The first time I heard this term, I laughed and thought, "How clever!"
But then I found out that other donors and donees, as well as scholars
like Tanya Cassidy (2012, 2014), refer to the promotion of breastfeeding,
breast milk nutrition, and the related practice of sharing milk (especially
against those who find sharing to be weird, dangerous, strange, or just
outright gross) as "lactivism."

Activisms

I have been describing the breast milk sharers as a heterarchical counternetwork of strange bedfellows that coalesces both in adherence to
and as a critique of institutional milk authorities, but this counternet-

work did not happen on its own. Lactivists have been instrumental in shaping how milk is shared.

To get at the (l)activism espoused by Jill, I am going to step back to examine the term "activism." First, activism suggests an exertion of agency. Both the meaning of milk and how it circulates are shaped by agents, even as lactivism is itself diverse and contested, with sharing seen as a social act with political ramifications undertaken with varying degrees of consciousness and strategizing.

Some sharers are simply acting in their own lives in accordance with their own private need, only accidentally serving as a model for others, if at all. This inadvertent activism by example (in the form of private actions, or what we might call microactivism) is not intended for public view, operates on a superlocal scale, and is far more serendipitous than organized grassroots activisms that address a public audience and seek to create change through protest, letter writing, or the consolidation of voting blocs. But private actions can also be potent and may enter into the arena of the overtly political. Microactivism can introduce milk sharing to sharers' families and friends, at times in spite of itself, and enhance the ability of public lactivists to shape the meaning of milk, and, therefore, attitudes about sharing.[2]

At the other extreme are militant milk activists, at times referred to by detractors as the "Breastapo," whose mission is to ensure that all babies are nourished with human milk as a human right and one that can even override a mother's freedom to choose how to feed her baby. A viable feminist critique of this position charges lactivists with undermining women's rights. Some mothers who were unable to provide sufficient milk complained to me that they had encountered hurtful or at least unwelcome pressure to breastfeed from friends or family and that some LLL leaders were "overly strict" or "not making sufficient allowances" for different bodies and family needs. Some women experienced this rigidity as an impossible contradiction, since they, according to LLL, are also not supposed to share.

Despite their antisharing stance, some women (like Jill) participated in LLL and in sharing (beyond the gaze of LLL leaders). For example, Mara and her partner, Selina, have two babies. Selina is a member of La Leche League, and while Mara and Selina know that the group does not approve of informal sharing, Mara explained that some members do it on the side. I mean they [LLL leaders] are *very* strict and the coordinator is a nurse and she believes that this is just extremely dangerous. So LLL is against this practice, maybe for legal reasons. And yes, it can be risky, but look at formula! For Selina, breastfeeding was all consuming in the beginning. She was not even sure that she wanted to breastfeed but because of health reasons and all that, but she said, "OK, I will do it," but for her it was very involved and complicated. She was in a lot of pain at first and had all kinds of problems, which is why she got involved with LLL in the first place. But, for her, it was also complicated in a gendered way, because she is more butch. But there was such pride in breastfeeding the baby! And we had a friend in LLL that was adopting, and she induced lactation and was eventually able to [do it], but Selina even donated to her.

Mothers may selectively accept advice, whether from LLL or friends and family, and thus parent in a way that fits their own worldviews and needs.

Within any society people view the world somewhat idiosyncratically and have different aptitudes for mobilizing their own or others' agency to effect change.[3] While some women may be inadvertent activists through private actions, we can think of activism as activity that intentionally, and rather self-consciously, works to bring about political or social change. The term implies a counterhegemonic intentionality, so when we hear "activist," we might identify hegemonic policy or activity being critiqued and then evaluate the alternative being offered.

Lactivists advance a probreastfeeding position: women should be able to breastfeed whenever and wherever they need to. Lactivists often consider breastfeeding, and by extension giving a child breast milk, a moral imperative. They may be critical of the formula industry and at times of mothers who choose formula. They work to promote breastfeeding awareness by explaining health benefits, educating people about laws related to breastfeeding, and working to strengthen policy that allows mothers to breastfeed in public and pump at work and that, in general, makes breastfeeding a normalized, protected aspect of life (rather than a hidden, sexualized, or embarrassing activity).

In a study of militant activism Charlotte Faircloth (2013) follows mothers who defy social norms by breastfeeding their children to "full term" (up to eight years of age) and practice a form of attachment parenting that requires them to forgo careers. This child-led practice is supported by what Faircloth recognizes as a choosy reading of biological, scientific, and even anthropological materials. In this context breastfeeding is mobilized as part of "intensive mothering," as identity work by mothers understood as moral citizens, where breastfeeding is framed as natural and normal, even as mothering is undersupported by the state, as is the case in the United States (especially in terms of maternity leave and child care) (Faircloth 2009). But lactivism in the United States has resulted in improved legislative protection for women pumping at work, and, when it is not forthcoming, women now have legal recourse.

For example, the American Civil Liberties Union (ACLU) and the Equal Employment Opportunity Commission brought a suit against a glass factory in Port Allegany, Pennsylvania, on behalf of Bobbi Bockoras.[4] Prior to giving birth Bockoras was one of only a few female machinists in a mostly male workforce. When she returned to work, the company, Saint-Gobain Verallia North America, asked her to pump in bathrooms and old locker rooms that she felt were unsanitary and insufficiently private. She was harangued by coworkers who brought her a bucket in an ill-conceived effort to compare her to a cow being milked and who covered the door handle of the room where she was pumping in grease and metal shards (acts that, according to an ACLU report [2013], her supervisor did not consider to be harassment). The suit asserts that the company failed to meet requirements of the 2010 Patient Protection and Affordable Care Act, which states that employers must "provide reasonable break time for an employee to express breast milk for her nursing child for one year after the child's birth each time such employee has need to express the milk. Employers are also required to provide a place, other than a bathroom, that is shielded from view and free from intrusion from coworkers and the public, which may be used by an employee to express breast milk" (U.S. Department of Labor 2010).[5]

The problem with the Affordable Care Act, lactivists argue, is that it applies only to companies with more than fifty employees and protects only hourly, not salaried, workers, instead of all working mothers.[6] So although lactivists still have work to do, the increasing visibility of breast milk and sharing is helping to challenge the squeamishness that underpins the discomfort that Bockoras's coworkers and employers allegedly experienced. This shift may ease women's ability to pump comfortably at work, especially if calls for pump designers to revamp the machines are heeded (see Martin and Cary 2014).

By engaging in a discursive battle to define access to milk as a human right, lactivists have been instrumental in shaping attitudes about breast milk, breastfeeding, and now sharing. This is important because the way we think of milk in the abstract, as a Peircian type, affects how we think about particular instances (tokens) of sharing.

The Abject

Because milk oozes from the postpartum body, it toggles between being sacred and profane and carries a heavy symbolic load. Sharing milk can thus be more than the distribution of a resource; it can become a highly charged interaction.

Orion explained that as soon as his family started looking for milk through Facebook and MilkShare

we found a medical doctor who became a regular donor for us. We also got a donor out at Ft. Stewart who just had many many gallons of milk. And then there was a tree farmer out in rural Georgia. And then, as a surprise, one of my colleagues at work's wife became a donor. He brought the bags to work, and would put them in the work fridge, which I am sure freaked a lot of people out. I would bring it home. So it was cool to us, but you know, to other people, breast milk is a bodily secretion, coming out of someone's breast! That's weird. I mean to find a breast secretion in your communal fridge? One time, I accidently [sic] left it overnight and the next day the principal, at our post-planning meeting, was like "be sure to clear stuff out of the fridge," and then she kind of gave a shiver, like an *eeeeuuuuwwww* shiver. I am pretty sure she was referring to the milk in there.

Orion's principal was responding to milk as an abject, bodily fluid. The milk is liminal: like other neither/nor secretions—menstrual blood, semen, sweat, excrement, and the placenta—milk is ambiguous, powerful, and subject to ritualized elaboration. Its power arises in part from the categorical ambiguity it poses: Is it self or not self? Is your semen, or menstrual blood, or excrement part of you or not? Is it sacred or profane? Or both? Or something in between?

As Mary Douglas (1966, 15) has pointed out, that which cannot be easily categorized leads to social anxiety, suppression, or avoidance: entities that fall between classificatory confines may be regarded as "polluting" or "dangerous." Douglas shows us how ambiguous things can seem threatening and become tabooed or domesticated through ritual. Postpartum purity rituals, or proscriptions about the type of breast milk to be given and when and where it can be given, function to protect categorical distinctions, which, because they are cultural, must be maintained through symbolic labor. Ideas about separating, purifying, demarcating, and punishing transgressions help to impose systems on an inherently untidy experience (Douglas 1996, 9). As a powerful liminal ooze, breast milk is implicated across a range of symbolic activities, from the rejection of the "beestings" (colostrum) in twentieth-century Britain (engorged breasts were relieved by another woman with a suckling glass, a puppy dog, or another, older child) (Fildes 1987; Hogan 2008), to Islamic milk-sibling kinship (Parkes 2005), to Ndembu puberty rituals (V. Turner 1967), to Sambian gender rites (Herdt 2005).

In the United States women's pregnant, postpartum, and lactating bodies are viewed as temporary (and liminal); the body is in a special phase with special rules and expectations and having attendant possibilities for pollution and power (Hogan 2008). Milk traverses the envelope of the skin, from inside the person to outside, bringing with it water, nutrients, and perhaps something more, troubling the easy congruence of personhood with bodily boundaries. And in fact there is a long history of the idea that breast milk might ferry personality, mood, or inclination to a recipient (not unlike the ways in which Lesley Sharp [2006] has shown that body organs are believed to bring with them traits of a heart, spleen, or kidney donor). Back in the eighteenth century, for example, Denis Diderot (1765) suggested that an acceptable wet nurse must be vigilant, wise, prudent, sweet, happy, gay, serious, and moderate in her penchant for love lest the baby be contaminated with a bad attitude.

A taboo against sharing because of the *something else* milk might bring with it shapes attitudes about allo-nursing and milk sharing.[7] I must admit that I found myself considering the possibility that a donor's personality might be carried in milk and tried to avoid getting "crazy-lady" milk by meeting mothers who were donating to us. The medical historian Susan Hogan (2008) notes in her work on the history of breastfeeding that a beloved friend demurred when Hogan offered to suckle her baby; knowing Hogan was healthy, this *something else* caused her friend discomfort. Allo-nursing today is still considered transgressive, something (for parents) to get used to. As one donor described her experience nursing a friend's baby, "it was a little weird at first, but after a while it was fine; [the baby] knew just what do to even though he had been on a bottle."

Exploring the effects of categorical ambiguity from a psychoanalytic perspective, Julia Kristeva (1982) defines the abject as a human reaction to a threatening breakdown in meaning caused by a disintegration between subject and object, or between self and other. An example of something that causes an abject reaction is the corpse, which reminds us of our own materiality; Kristeva points to other objects that elicit a similar reaction: wounds, excrement, sewage, or even the skin that forms on the surface of warm milk. I know that I experience a thrilling sense of disgust when faced with warm milk skin and thus am drawn to it. I have the same reaction of nausea combined with acute fascination when I see hair on a shower drain. I think this subjective texturing is what Kristeva (1982, 9) was getting at when she associated the abject with *jouissance*: "One does not know it, one does not desire it, one joys in it [*on en jouit*]. Violently and painfully. A passion."

But drain hair and milk skin are after the fact: from the perspective of psychoanalysis the abject marks a moment of mother-child separation, when the boundary between self and other (me versus mother) solidifies. The abject marks a boundary condition. Mother's milk sends us to an important site of abjection, which is why it is viewed as sacred, polluting, gross, magical, and so forth. Its abject nature makes it ripe for artistic and social projects whose goals range from adventurous titillation to political critique to collaborative world-making.

This is why even pondering the possibility of sharing elicits reactions in some people. When Kaya was considering donation, she was surprised by how many people she talked with "seemed put off by it. Even grossed out! I mean, when I was coming along, moms would just share their milk if there was another baby around, so I guess I just did not think it was a big deal."

Some of my friends had similar reactions. Carrie, who had given birth to her first child when we started receiving milk, told me that after she saw us sharing and found herself unable to keep up with her baby's needs, she too had decided to become a donee. Describing her first donor experience, she admitted, "I didn't know how it would be. I thought it would be so weird. I had seen yours [donated milk in our fridge] and it totally freaked me out! I thought, 'Now, that it is disgusting!' I had brought some club soda over to your house and I didn't want [the bottles] to touch it. But then, when I had Lacy and understood, all of a sudden, [milk] became this amazing thing. But now I wonder what people think when they see milk in my freezer. It's a Hollywood comedy to drink breast milk in your coffee!"

And she is right, because breast milk, like other body fluids, is seldom seen and rarely described or pictured in popular culture. So when it does show up, its power is exploited to produce laughter or other affective states.

In her exegetical essay "From 'Gift to Loss' to Self Care" Fiona Giles (2010) examines the abject power of milk in contemporary film. She describes how films such as *Les valseuses* (1974) (which contains an adult nursing scene) use milk to provoke an abject reaction, while other films use milk for comedic ends, such as *Look Who's Talking* (1989) or *Me, Myself & Irene* (2000), both of which play on a character's revulsion at the idea of accidentally drinking breast milk. Giles (2010, 236) argues that these films reflect an unresolved and underexplored cultural fascination with breast milk and the capacity of women to lactate; this fascination is expressed in cinema as the interplay of the erotic and the abject, of desire and disgust.

Giles goes on to suggest that lactation and breastfeeding exist along a continuum of embodied care for both adults and children to be viewed as a part of our sexuality, as suggested by *A Place on Earth* (*Mesto na zemle* [2001]), in which a hippie commune in Moscow offers breastfeeding as sustenance to a homeless population, as well as by the Japanese black comedy *Visitor Q* (2001). *Visitor Q* is remarkable because it comes full circle, linking what might be construed as a shocking scene (of a mother breastfeeding her grown children and husband) to venerated traditions we see expressed in Renaissance paintings, Greco-Roman mythology, and Shinto Buddhism. Here lactation is shown simultaneously as care, wholeness, power, and female sensuality.

I would not necessarily expect to find many examples of *Visitor Q*-like scenes in mainstream American society, but I was surprised by the rarity of breast milk in contemporary visual culture since many well-known artists, such as Méret Oppenheim, Günter Brus, Rudolf Schwarzkogler, Karen Finley, Kiki Smith, Joseph Beuys, Mona Hatoum, Robert Gober, and two of my personal favorites, Bob Flanagan and Joel-Peter Witkin, do work with the abject. There was even an exhibition in 1993 at the Whitney Museum, *Abject Art: Repulsion and Desire in American Art*, and another at the Tate in 1995, *Rites of Passage: Art for the End of a Century*, both of which were inspired by Kristeva's work. But despite the references to breastfeeding in paintings by popular, modern artists such as Frida Kahlo (e.g., *My Nurse and I* [1937] or *Love Embrace of the Universe* [1949]) or Wolfgang Herzig (e.g., *Judith I* [1966]), mothers who post photographs of themselves breastfeeding their own babies can be reported for indecency on social media, even on the HM4MB Facebook site through which many donations are made.

Despite all of the press about the joys of breastfeeding and benefits of milk, both are still viewed as out of bounds. The lactating woman is leaking, excessive, dangerous, and polluting, and so is her milk. In exploring this idea the artist Jess Dobkin staged *The Lactation Station Breast Milk Bar* in 2006 at the Ontario College of Art and Design. As one scholarly commentator put it, her work "forces us to confront the judgmental, suspicious gaze that we project on women's bodies, particularly the bodies of breastfeeding women" (Van Esterik 2009, 23). Lactivists frame this same potency as positive and empowering, reclaiming the lactating breast from a judgmental and/or sexualized gaze. In this vein Lynn Randolph's painting *Venus* is accompanied by an essay defending spectacular lactation as a form of resistance to the policing of women's bodies such as that exerted on Facebook.

Randolph (2010) writes that Venus is "not a Goddess in the classical sense of the contained figure, she is an unruly woman, actively making a spectacle of herself, queering Botticelli, leaking, projecting, shooting milk, transgressing the boundaries of her body, Botticelli's shell has been turned upside down, and it is raining. Hundreds of years have passed since Botticelli painted his Venus and we are still engaged in a struggle for interpretive power over our bodies in a society where they are marked as a battleground by the church and state in legal and medical skirmishes." She articulates, in words and in paint, ideas that reverberated in my interviews, as women like Issa described women's bodies as sites of political struggle and pointed out that sharing challenges the disciplining of women's bodies by a predominantly male medical establishment.

The Refusal to Abdicate

Although not everyone was as explicit as Issa, her meditation on sharing echoed others' sentiments. Formerly a Russian-language translator for the American government, Issa is now a doula and an active member of my local counternetwork. She strategically promotes women's health, helps women gain access to information, and brings support services related to health, pregnancy, and childcare to those who cannot afford them. A grandmother herself, she is older than the childbearing donors and donees that make up most of the community. Well known locally, Issa was instrumental in helping us get linked into the community. She explained to me, "Back when I was a new mom, we did something like this. We did a lot of cross nursing, but it was all family and friends. But these Facebook circles and so forth, just expand our community phenomenally."

As Issa pointed out, there is a lot more to sharing than spreading resources. Sharing can also make community. She identified a radical altruism that confounds the logic of the commodity market, medical authority, and the materialist interpretation of milk. "This is pure generosity," she said. "It's a woman thing. And you know I'm big on women! When a lot of women do things together, something happens. To me, it seems like there is a lot of pride in participating in what in more traditional times would have taken place in other circles, in tribes or families,

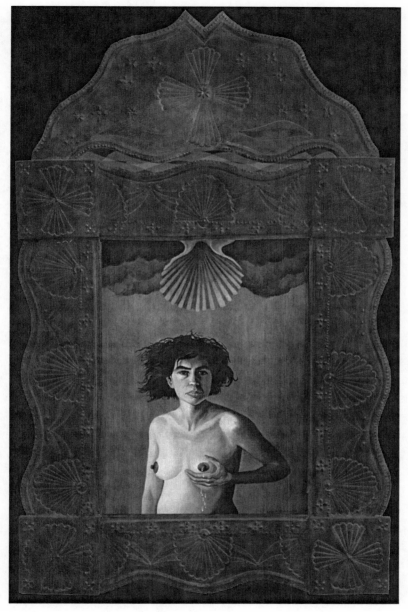

22. Lynn Randolph, *Venus*, 1992. Oil on board. Collection of the National Museum of Women in the Arts, Washington DC. Image used by permission of the artist.

but this is a different kind of community, more faceless or unknown, but this highlights the altruism that is at work, maybe it is altruism at its highest." Sharing that exceeds the production of kin and friend for a faceless community is performative and may entail few if any future expectations but still give back in terms of pleasure and satisfaction.

Milk donation is somewhat costly to donors in terms of time, labor, and emotional investment. But as Issa put it,

> it is important to highlight the aspect of altruism. A lot of social movements start with that because people want to give, to give back, to help. And the feeling of doing that is off the scale! I mean co-nursing is like that, and if we would have done milk storing and sharing [in my day], it would have been a great feeling. But that was not even on our radar! We never even conceived of such a thing! Or we would have done it. You have to remember, I was living in Boston in the 1960s and 70s where experimental community living was big. If we could have done it, we all would have been like, "Hell yeah, you should have some of my awesome milk!"

Besides pride, there is a dynamic politics implied in the way Issa links sharing to communal experiments critical of mainstream society. Altruism is a historically constructed idea about human potential that is usually defined as a concern for the well-being of others with whom one may or may not have an ongoing social relationship. In breast milk sharing, as in the communes in which Issa lived, altruistic donors bypass the principle of economic self-interest foundational to American capitalism.

Even though anthropologists have fatally critiqued the notion of "rational man," he continues to haunt economic, psychological, and sociological theory. The very idea that one might act selflessly for the benefit of others runs so counter to the way people are thought to behave that there are serious academic debates about whether or not altruism is even possible. Much of this debate in anthropology takes place in evolutionary studies that consider whether altruism as an adaptation may confer advantage either at the level of the individual (the level upon which natural selection is usually thought to operate), where it may be selected for if it increases the probability of survival of close relatives (Relethford 2012), or at the level of the group ("eusociality"), where altruism may be costly to an individual but benefit the group (Wilson 2012, 2013).

In writing about how motivation is presented in the social sciences Richard Wilk (1993) argues that decision making is classified into three categories—economic, social, or moral—but they are not mutually exclusive; he shows that in fact these categories are folk models of the explanations that people use to describe their actions. And indeed we must take seriously the fact that sharers highlight how giving and receiving takes place among strangers not only outside of the market but also beyond kinship or even friendship, and they use the term "altruism" to describe and explain what they are doing. It has all three components: moral, social, and economic.

The for-profit milk and formula market presses against this landscape of "altruistic" donation by offering alternatives. As Issa put it, "of course, labs try to reproduce the effects of breast milk, or try to make breast milk–like formulas. This is what is so paradoxical, yet so American! Why trust a woman's body when you can control a chemically formulated version? This is exactly how men took over the birthing from midwives. It [the hospital birthing process] is presented as all clean and controlled and spic and span. So we have generosity, altruism, and love—which is the essence of birthing and having babies—versus a sanitized, profitable, hospital environment, that is usually for, let's face it, men—and I hate to say that! But usually it is, and it is offered as 'safe' to make it seem better, or more attractive."

Obliquely referring to the dangers conjured to justify scientific, sanitized, medicalized scenarios, she continued, "But babies and also mothers sometimes do die. And that *is* sad, but it is also a part of life, part of the organic nature of life that you cannot always control. But when you introduce 'safety' into [lab-made or treated] breast milk to appease fears about life, it works as an enticement, and takes milk out of an understanding of it as something coming from the earthly, natural body and into the realm of the spic and span, squeaky [clean] lab. And really it is a provocation, because it appeals to the notion of risk." Issa is offering a view of life that embraces, even celebrates, the gambles associated with living. Her perspective is the polar opposite of neoliberalized mothering in which there is an effort to eradicate every conceivable risk.

The hidden costs of capitulating to a spic-and-span, technologized milk distribution refract an ethics of life. What does it mean to have and to be given responsibility for another life? What does it mean to live with, to commune with others? What activities and practices do we extend, or retract, in creating the warp and weft of society? How can we live, and die, well? Ideas advanced by lactivists like Issa run parallel to those of scholars who like Donna Haraway (1998, 2013) valorize but also critique science, explore different ways to live better together, and forge liberatory spaces by recognizing that to be alive is to take risks together.

Milk sharers discuss risk and how to use science and technology to share well. In talking about tips suggested by social media sites we both used, Melanie told me that she was "always impressed by people's willingness to give out their milk, and to share their medical records. I usually asked, but there were times when I just took their word for [their good health]. I can't say that I felt great about that, but it's what we did." Her face and body language suggested that she felt sheepish admitting this, but she seemed to feel better when I confessed that we had at times done the same: trusted.

This trust is the flip side of risk, which, as Alphonso Lingis (2004, ix, original emphasis) tells us in his investigations of traveling, constitutes human connection:

> Every day we deal with people who occupy posts in an established social system where behaviors are socially defined and sanctioned. . . . But to *trust you* is to go beyond what I know and to hold on to the real individual that is you. . . . When we leave our home and community to dwell awhile in some remote place, it happens every day that we trust a stranger, someone with whom we have no kinship bonds, no common loyalty to a community or creed, no contractual obligations. . . . We attach to someone whose words or whose movements we do not understand, whose reasons or motives we do not see. Our trust short-circuits this space . . . and makes contact with the real individual agent there—with *you*.

Trust sets up a foundation for connection, but alone it does not explain one of the most significant payoffs of milk sharing, which is to illuminate how to better *live with*.

As a phenomenologist Lingis takes us into the arena of the subjective by describing trust as "the most joyous kind of bond with another living being. . . . It takes courage to trust someone you do not know. There is an exhilaration in trusting that builds on itself. . . . Indeed, just as there is courage in trust, so there is pleasure, exhilaration in trust: trust laughs at dangers. . . . Trust is courageous, giddy, and lustful" (2008, x, xii). The stranger work in milk sharing is exhilarating in a deeply existential way, because sharing opens the possibility for new ways of being together. Strangers are risking, trusting, being together at a critical point, in the reproduction of care and life, at a place where the sacred and the abject are united. Sharers leap into the unknowable together, which is why milk sharing is experienced at times as emotional, cathartic, and loving. So how do people make decisions about whom to trust when they travel or share? In exploring this theme Issa said what most sharers know:

There are always risks . . . which are minimal in the big picture. But a lot of times bringing up risk will play into the fears people have and to the idea of "being a good mother." But that's capitalism, and advertising. On the other side, women instinctively have an intuition, and a lot of times it kicks in when you become a mother, and of course you can be wrong or mistaken, but usually, whatever you *feel* is powerful, and that can work against the technological, squeaky-clean lab approach, and, really, I see it working a lot of times as an issue of empowerment. The squeaky-clean, controlled lab approach tries to strip away the validity of intuition as a form of knowledge. But there is a lot riding on it; so questions like "Is that really a good idea?" or "Is that safe?" can get people to second-guess the choices they have made based on deep feelings, and whether we trust [those feelings] or some other way of knowing, it is a personal thing. Look, we all want the best for our children, and there are many ways of knowing. Intuitive skills *are* real skills that help us decide, for example, if this or that environment is right for this child. And these skills are, well not explicitly, but they are, let's say *undermined* by a more technological approach. It's not a conspiracy, but it is a power play by folks who think they know better, who think that intuitive wisdom is not valid. But science and intuition are not mutually exclusive! Knowledge comes in many forms. And that's OK, because everyone has to do what they think is right at the time, but [being the person to] question authority and ask questions can be challenging.

In questioning the hierarchy of scientific over intuitive knowledge making and calling for the situational deployment of decision-making skills, Issa validates both. Milk sharing is not a rejection or dismissal of science or technology but rather a calculated, embodied engagement with it. This is why I found doctors, lactation consultants, and LLL members sharing milk but giving the caveat that personal sharing is different from their professional recommendations and obligations.

Amber, for example, is deeply involved with the science of breast-feeding and breast milk. As a board certified lactation consultant she knows as well as anyone the risks of sharing identified by science, but as a donee she did not get any paperwork from any of her donors, explaining, "Not from my sister. Not from my friend (I mean we had an informal conversation, and I knew she was healthy), and not from my other three donors with whom I had very little contact. I just trusted the lactation consultant that connected us. And, I mean if you can't trust an OB [one of her donors was an obstetrician], who can you trust?"

But as Amber explained, the stakes were different when the tables were turned and she became a milk donor. She had approached her donee about testing:

[I asked her] if she wanted documents, and I would have been happy to get tests and provide her with anything she wanted, but she said no. So, I went online, printed out a questionnaire and filled it out. I gave that to her. I felt like I wanted to provide that. But, the main issue is that this is donation. When money gets involved, there has to be testing, and documentation, because motivations are different: people might say, hey I can add some milk or water or whatever, so I see that as a really important distinction. One mom to another is different. Me? I went with intuition. On the whole, people do this with a good heart, a full heart, and there is nothing to hide. I felt fine doing paperwork as a donor, but as a donee, I needed the milk and felt that it was the right thing, so I took it without paperwork. And mom-to-mom sharing is a beautiful thing.

So as a mother Amber has been both a donor and a donee, but as a professional she does not and cannot recommend it "because of the liability." Pointing out the contradiction, she explained that "there are not a lot of lactation consultants that know about my sharing activities. There is a stigma there. I think a lot of my colleagues would support it, but many would see it as a big, big risk. But there are personal feelings and then there are professional responsibilities—it's the liability issue." So, yes, Issa is right, questioning authority is challenging; the solution for Amber has been to cleave her private from her public face. Professional words and deeds support the policy, and authority, of the International Lactation Consultant Association establishment, largely for financial reasons; in her personal life she quietly upends it.

Perhaps we should not be surprised about the use of the body in these unsanctioned ways since women's bodies have long been a site for resistance to patriarchal authority. In *Holy Feast and Holy Fast* Caroline Walker Bynum (1987) describes how the medieval body was wielded by women, perhaps because it was all they had to work with. Bynum writes persuasively against a long-held position that fasting women were anorexics to suggest that, although a version of anorexia may have been at play, fasting must be considered in a larger context, and that larger context was food. Food was the arena of women, they were expected to produce it and serve it, and it also had a heightened religious or at least spiritual significance. To eat or not eat was to exert authority, or at least power, in this domain.

In our own society food preparation remains women's work—and the act of nourishing one's own baby in addition to others' works as a performance of successful motherhood, an index of fecundity, and an avenue for feeling fulfilled and empowered. For sharers, making and sharing milk is a sacred act that would be sullied by commodification. Sharing is a quiet but unequivocal refusal to behave according to the mandates of health officials or to the logic of capitalism. These ordinary women (and men) are occupying the interstices of public places (the Internet, LLL meetings, and parents' groups) to counterhegemonic ends. But what kinds of politics inhere in these acts? What kind of (l) activism is this?

An Ordinary Friendly Act

In *Life as Politics* Asef Bayat (2010) describes the appropriation of space and utilities by marginalized third-world urbanites in the Middle East and indeed all over the developing world. While some have looked at the marketing of fruits and vegetables in public streets or the sale of cell phone minutes on corners as poor people's survival strategies or tactics of urban social movements, Bayat's work highlights their creative, strategic expansion. His notion of "quiet encroachment" describes the silent and protracted but pervasive advancement of ordinary people in the space of the propertied and powerful, and the larger public, in order to survive and improve their lives; these activities are marked by largely atomized and prolonged mobilizations with episodic collective action, characterized by open and fleeting struggles without clear leadership, ideology, or structured organization (Bayat 2010, 56).

Quiet encroachment is not explicit political activity but acts performed by dispersed individuals and families for the purpose of acquiring basic necessities. People tapping electrical lines or water pipes in Cairo or Tehran are emblematic of quiet encroachment. Bayat developed this idea out of his observations of subaltern responses to globalization, with its simultaneous consequence of increased integration with greater social exclusion and informalization in the Muslim Middle East, but he wonders if it might have relevance for other third-world places. For my part, though it may appear to be a strange, even unwarranted comparison at first, I find it relevant in relation to my observations about first-world, middle-class milk sharers, as milk sharing is an individualized act that shifts milk and trust into the realm of the political. So how might this work?

Going back to Marx's contested depiction of the *Lumpenproletariat*, Bayat tracks the history of sociological scholarship on the marginalized poor. In explicating the experience, role, and future of the "underclass," he shows how scholars have debated issues of class agency, consciousness, stability, and revolutionary potential. Rather than rehearse the full debate on the politics of the poor (which Bayat sees coalescing into four major perspectives: the passive poor, survival strategies, urban territorial movement, and everyday resistance models), I extract three aspects of the debate about underclass activism for a discussion about the politics of milk sharing: power, network, and intentionality.

What about power? When we think about strategic responses to structural circumstances, we can consider everyday practices as well as organized resistance. Gramsci and Foucault helped pave the way for looking at resistance like this when they identified power as not only decentered and circulating but as distributed along particular trajectories with a tendency to accumulate in sites that advance class interests (which is why, capillary as power may be, the state and other authoritative institutions must be examined with care [Bayat 2010, 54]). To wield power, or to become empowered, subalterns may create, or seek opportunities within a moral economy (relying on trust, reciprocity, or voluntarism) using social power (for example, free time, social skills, or networking), with the household as a central unit of production of livelihood (Friedmann 1992). These opportunities may be discovered, or produced, within "free spaces" (Woods 1993), political or social interstices, gray areas of the law, or spaces beyond easy surveillance. As micropolitics, third-world urban subaltern action under these conditions tends to be spatialized and local, with the potential for a great deal of variation in individual perspectives; this form of resistance is thus flexible, small scale, and unbureaucratic (Bayat 2010, 52)—in other words, heterarchical.

Milk sharing is undertaken within a moral economy using social power by a shifting, markedly unbureaucratic group. Part of the reason that this sharing community is in flux is that donors' ability to give and donees' needs change rather dramatically over the course of a year or so. What's more, exchanges tend to be local, in part defined by the distance one can comfortably drive with an infant in tow (usually within a three- to four-hour radius) or how long milk will remain frozen solid using low technology (ice and a cooler).

But how might lactivism and milk sharing as quiet encroachment support or undermine the state or other authoritative institutions? As part of a growing informal economy it flies in the face of state surveillance of commodity production and exchange, the profit motive necessary to the smooth functioning of capitalism, and social demands to acquiesce to a hierarchy of knowledge that privileges science, documentation, and policy developed by authoritative institutions. Milk sharing takes place between single individuals, so it is virtually invisible to the state, is outside of any regulation or mandate (or protection) by the law, and bypasses formal markets for both human milk and formula. It takes place outside of milk banks and for-profit corporations, eschewing existing attempts to capture milk circulating through sharing, which are already under way by both types of institutions since demand by insured customers for products from banks and for-profits companies far outweighs supply. Sharers' refusal to commodify milk thus represents a challenge to the state, whose very existence is predicated on the extraction of capital from all forms of production.

So even if it is not a social movement per se, milk sharing is activist in that sharers support a heterarchical counternetwork forged out of a biocultural condition (lack of sufficient milk) combined with a political, ideological, and/or emotional impetus.[8] Participants as a group do not have a clear allegiance to either left- or right-wing politics; in fact the group is populated by strange bedfellows, at least in terms of basic political orientations, and does have a markedly doubled character as both local and international.[9]

But what about intention? The communities Bayat describes—those who tap water or electricity—may not be acting out of an intentional resistance but out of need, though their actions may lead to welcome changes in urban infrastructure or governance. Within the sharing community, women, especially those who called themselves "(l)activists," such as Issa and Jill, were clear about their participation in sharing as a critique of authoritative institutions, while others saw it as simply "helping out" a baby or another mother.

We might sever activism from the activist as a heuristic move to identify actions that result in social change. Milk sharing as (l)activism, even undertaken by those who do not claim an explicitly activist identity, has a transformative effect in that it is a form of doing, of making, of being in the world. It is a de facto enunciation of an alternative value and economic system that not only does not cooperate with (if not outright opposes) hegemonic authority but can engender a feeling of thrilling delight, experienced as tears and expressions of thanks, love, and relief, that asks to be comprehended as *communitas*, even if fleeting or sporadic.

I use the term "communitas" to underscore how sharers come together not only sociopolitically but phenomenologically: sharing, as well as the trust it entails, is an experience that, as the rapper Rich Homie Quan says, makes "you feel some type of way."[10] Within anthropology the term "communitas" was developed by Victor Turner, who adopted it from the anarchist Paul Goodman (Rohrer 2013, 83). Turner (1967, 1969) renders communitas as a feeling or experience of collective solidarity, of one-ness, as opposed to divisive individuality, that emerges in anti-structure, often within the context of ritual. In a related comment on what makes anthropology unique, Lingis (2007, 78) writes that fieldwork sets the anthropologist apart from other kinds of social scientists: "Government officials, traders, explorers, and missionaries are also in the field, and longer. Is it not the heady, intoxicating, unforgettable abandon to trust that makes the anthropologist's experience so distinctive?" This giddy, even quasi-erotic trust is, I think, what Edith Turner (2011, 4) is also getting at in *Communitas: The Anthropology of Collective Joy*, where she expands the notion of communitas to "togetherness itself" to elucidate the affective qualities of communitas as part of the fieldwork experience.

Recalling the work of Goodman, the Turners, and Lingis, I know that as a participant-observer I experienced at times an intoxicating joy in a deep attachment to a stranger bucking authority with me. Our donors seemed just as energized by the partnership, at times thanking *me* with enthusiasm.

Here a one-ness is somewhat imaged, and, unlike the kind of unity we might expect to note within traditional rites of passage where initiates move together in time and space to experience communitas, the digital technology that makes milk sharing possible creates a kind of (paradoxically) asynchronic communitas that is egalitarian (at least in theory), decentralized, informally organized, organic, aleatory, localized while globalized, and marked by idiosyncrasy. In contrast milk banks and formula offer standardized experience and a standardized product, through formal, rational channels. Of course not everyone experiences communitas, nor would they do so all of the time. But in this version of milk sharing—even if communitas may be an exception and not the rule—it does represent an affective variation experienced by participants.

Admittedly, a counterhegemonic bent was not articulated by all participants, and some shares are rather pragmatic, devoid of affective expressiveness. So what does this tell us about the role of agency? Identifying political intentionality in the domestic activities of middle-class (sub)urbanites in the American South is tricky, since being overtly political, much less activist, is largely frowned upon. In the case of milk sharing the willingness and ability to describe sharing as a manifestation of resistance is varied, but I did find a clear inclination to claim membership in an imaginary community of sharers (both men and women), which is akin to what I think Bayat is describing with his idea of a "passive network"—a group of individuals who are mobilized to act collectively when their accomplishments are challenged by an authority such as the state or other institution (e.g., La Leche League, the American Academy of Pediatrics, or private companies attempting to disrupt sharing through commodification or criticism).

The mobilization of a passive network is never a given, but I see glimmers of a more organized demand for milk as a human right as researchers, critics, and milk banks contest sharing. Breast milk advocates and milk bank representatives, like staff at the South Carolina Milk Bank, hope that one day human milk will become available to all babies as a universal right, like access to water, housing, and antiretroviral drugs should be today. All of this must be balanced against parents' rights to decide what is appropriate for them and for their children, but there are already activists discussing the right to breast milk, "based on the right to life, to adequate nutrition and to the highest attainable standard of health, and based on women's rights, which includes the right to breastfeed, to breastfeeding education and to paid maternity leave" (Ball 2010).[11] Taking this approach even further, participants at the 2012 World Breastfeeding Conference in Delhi called upon all to adopt "a human right-based approach to the protection, promotion and support

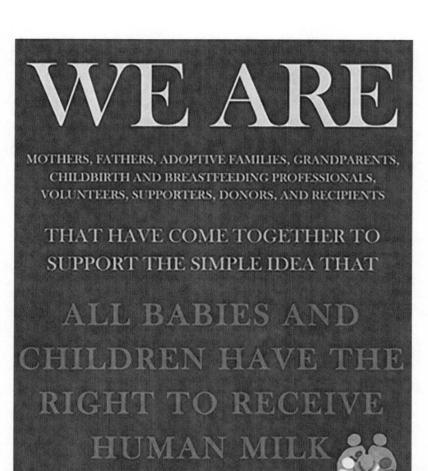

23. "We Are" poster on HM4HB.net. Courtesy of HM4HB and Stephanie Benelli.

of breastfeeding and infant and young child feeding at international, national, sub-national and community levels."[12] In May 2014 (just four years after it was founded), the Human Milk 4 Human Babies Facebook page for Georgia expressed the position that all babies and children have the right to receive human milk, stopping just short of claiming that it should be viewed as a right on par with shelter, health care, and freedom from violence. At the moment, they are very likely preaching to the choir.

Galactivism

There is a danger in seeing resistance everywhere. An alternative would be to distinguish the kind of resistance enacted by, for instance, gossip, from actions that make one vulnerable to physical or mental harm, arrest, or even death. Keeping in mind the importance of maintaining the distinctions of intensity that mark various acts of resistance, we can compare milk sharing with the struggles of third-world subalterns without constituting a dangerous and "savage leveling that diminishes rather than intensifies our sensitivities to injustice" (Brown 1996, 730).

Bayat points out that even privileged segments of the developing world may resort to quiet encroachment as they are squeezed by advanced neoliberal governance, and I would note that these are the same politics squeezing the American middle class through a combination of flat wage-earning power, a reconfiguration of the global labor market, and the defanging of unions. In these ways the milk-sharing community, peopled by a shifting cast of middle-class parents, has something in common with the groups Bayat describes in that sharers are exploiting a legal blank zone. Sharing, considered illicit by some, is not illegal. But as industry treats milk as an ever more valuable resource, it is placed squarely into the realm of political economy, with milk management taking on a distinctly biopolitical tang.

In a study of water infrastructure in Mumbai, Nikhil Anand (2011) tracks the intersection of technologies of politics and the politics of technology to describe what he calls "hydraulic citizenship," which has everything to do with who can get how much water to flow where, given their geophysical location, network of relations, and available tools and technologies. Unlike water, the flow of milk is viewed by the state, for the moment anyway, as a private matter, and thus the state has little to say about it. On the other hand, with so many powerful institutions, including federal ones, insisting that breast milk is best, it is surprising that activists have not pressured the state to ensure milk availability as a right of citizenry. Sharing poses the question: what might a (ga)lactic citizenship look like?

Sharing, as a pattern of social interaction, is of particular interest since American culture is shaped by capitalism. As a successful heterarchical social practice that critiques it, milk sharing may contain object lessons. What impact will this "hit-and-run" critical practice have on capitalism? How is capitalism responding? And why does it matter? As sharing becomes more visible, questions about commodification loom ever larger.

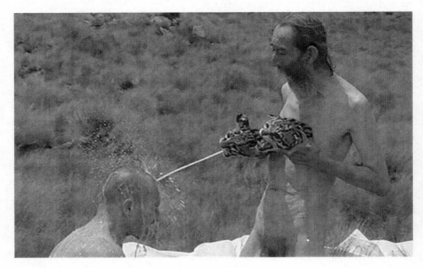

24. Film still from *Holy Mountain* (1973).

Holy Mountains

On his way to a costume party in Paris, Alejandro Jodorowsky found a faux cheetah tail in a garbage can and attached it to his rear. That night he met several surrealists with whom he would become intimately connected.

Soon after, Maurice Chevalier came to find him in a car with cheetah-skin seats, which Jodorowsky took as a sign. During the next several decades he learned from other masters besides Chevalier, such as Ejo Takata, Erich Fromm, Pachita (a Mexican sorceress), Carlos Castaneda, the artist Topor, and the playwright Fernando Arrabel. Each pushed Jodorowsky in his search for the spiritual knowledge he has inserted in work that is meant to touch, transform, and change the audience.[1]

In his capacities as a director, screenwriter, playwright, actor, author, producer, tarot card reader, and composer, Jodorowsky has demonstrated an ambivalent attitude toward art as commodity, leaving the sale of his work to others and proclaiming, "I have always had a horror of business matters. When someone presents me with a contract, I do not discuss it; I can't even stand to read it all. . . . I have lived this way without a problem" (Jodorowsky 2009, 72). Being rich is being free to create.

His film *Holy Mountain* (1973), a hallucinogenic romp through the modern search for enlightenment, peels back layer after layer of ideological illusion: religion, the state, war, beauty, film, the self, and so forth. The lactating breast scene pictured here was restaged in 2010 by A-list editorial photographer Mario Sorrenti for the New York issue of *V 67*. There in glossy color, a sexy model, Natasha Poly, shoots milk from jaguar breasts onto a naked man (see Sauers 2010). Although one gets a sense of Sorrenti's admiration, this postmodern citation practice—all image, no content—is distinctly commercial and works well in juxtaposition with Jodorowsky's critique of the commodity. This image in fact would not be bad on a box of milk.

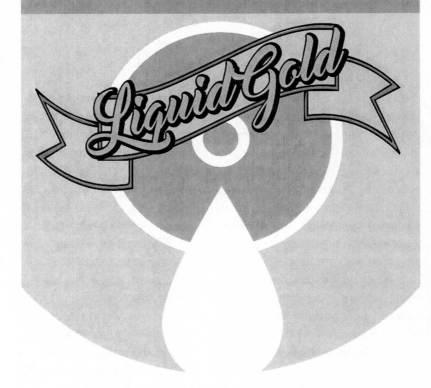

25. Zteven Zangbang, layout for *Ad for Liquid Gold–Humilk*, 2015.
Courtesy of the artist.

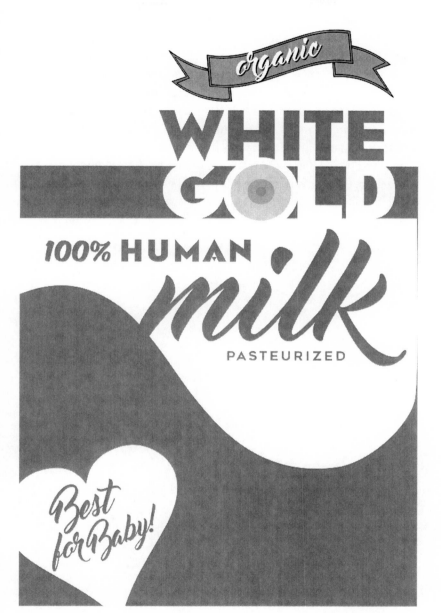

26. Zteven Zangbang, layout for *Ad for White Gold*, 2015. Courtesy of the artist.

Nell pulled six-month-old Mary out of her car seat and stuffed her into a Moby Wrap before zipping quickly through the Whole Foods parking lot to avoid the rain. Inside she selected three gorgeous pears out of an artfully balanced pyramid and placed them in her cart, adding squash, kale, and sweet potato, all organic. Rounding the corner, she noticed that the breast milk area had been relocated to the frozen nutritionals section. Stopping to examine a new brand, she considered how well Mary had done with Pamalat's A Mother's Love and Nobisco's less expensive Chubby Baby product. She saw that the Holy Mountains brand White Gold, Organic was back. Nell checked her wallet, then grabbed all of the boxes left on the shelf, wondering how long the shortage would continue.

5   Economic Matters

Breast milk, that most ancient and fundamental of nourishments, is
becoming an industrial commodity, and one of the newest frontiers
of the biotechnology industry.

ANDREW POLLACK, *New York Times*, March 20, 2015

When I was learning about sharing, I found out that breast milk was
undergoing a process of commodification. By mid-2012 a few potential
donors had suggested that we purchase their milk. This situation presented a quandary: I could see that these women needed money, but
buying milk went against community standards. Then again, was I
exploiting my donors? Is a buying relationship really all that different?
Shouldn't they be compensated?

Breast milk and its various simulated and synthetic counterparts are
subject to the processes of commodity capitalism, but the process does
not go uncontested.[2] Debates about whether and how to commodify,
regulate, or oversee milk are entertained by sharers and increasingly by
those representing scientific, governmental, and corporate institutions.

We know that capitalism must continuously seek new markets. It
requires us to find ways to extract or translate life itself into capital; the
contemporary form of this practice is known as biocapitalism (see Helmreich 2008). The patenting of genes is but one example. A refusal to
participate in the commodification of milk by insisting on donation,
rejecting the reduction of life to capital, constitutes a resistance to biocapitalism. Both donating and commodifying milk can be understood
in this context.

Algebras of Value

Gifting is a highly ritualized, culturally specific activity. As opposed to the way many societies view the gift, Americans tend to view a gift with strings attached as not a real gift. We tend to define it somewhat idealistically: it should be neither in return for a previous gift nor in anticipation of a future recompense. The recipient should not perceive it as an exchange that requires repayment, nor should the giver view it in terms of a reciprocal cycle.

What functions might the gifting of breast milk have? Is not the act of indebting, and of accepting the debt, the crux of the matter when it comes to gifting? Certainly replacing bags or giving someone vitamins for their donation might discount it as an act of disinterested exchange, but it does not rise to the level of barter or sale since there are no explicit terms, temporal expectations, or punishments for failure to comply. Mothers say they would give milk without receiving anything in return: I was told on numerous occasions that items I offered were appreciated but not required or even desired.

Marcel Mauss (2016) posits that the difference between a commodity and a gift has to do with the kind of expectations people have as a result of participating in an exchange.[3] The strings attached to a gift, rather than being reviled as self-serving or sneaky, might be celebrated as an index of trust: the strings attached are like outstretched hands, reaching out to a receiver who has the power to accept (or reject) them. This metaphorical linking of hands constitutes the warp and weft of a community.

These connections are not just niceties but necessary to the functioning of a society so thoroughly entrenched in market activity, like that of the United States. Gifts, even of things acquired through purchase, tend to operate with such high degrees of social salience that I frankly have to wonder if a market economy could exist without a gifting foundation underneath it to underscore common interests and futures.

Many of our belongings are acquired through purchase with no, or virtually no, implied future obligations, and while these purchases do make dense contributions to the reproduction of political and economic dynamics, they contribute less to personal relationships. Breast milk sharing, insofar as it takes place between willing families, does have the benefit of weaving a community together.

When we accepted milk, our "debt" was nebulous: it seemed to contain a commitment to care, to good parenting, and to community making. Donors redirected talk when I offered them milk bags or flowers or children's books. Karen told me, for example, "Thank you, but I just think it is so wonderful that you are taking all of this time to give your baby what he needs," and Elsa said, "We [moms] have to stick together and help each other out." At first I was confused by these remarks, but eventually I realized that some donors were more concerned about the meanings of the gift than with recompense, which was appreciated but superfluous.

The movement of milk from a lactating mom to another family corresponds with an anthropological notion of the gift, insofar as, unlike a market transaction, it creates and maintains social relationships. Even when my sister gave us milk, it benefited my child, but, and perhaps what is more important, it made visible and strengthened our kinship ties.

Gifting also has a temporal dimension. How much time should pass before you give something back? There is a delayed response, and how much time passes until the responsive act is culturally variable. When my sister gave us milk, there was no request or expectation of immediate or near-term reward. But as partners in a long-standing reciprocal relationship, we often give to each other. Breast milk slid rather easily into the back-and-forth movement of shoes, gossip, books, jewelry, and favors that has been taking place all of our lives.

Of course different conditions apply in stranger-to-stranger shares. When there is an immediate return (in the form of bags, flowers, or other items), it might begin to look like a barter, a less socially charged transaction. But these relationships are not cut and dried; they may fall anywhere on a continuum. One donor asks for a swaddling blanket or set of teething rings. Another pumps five to ten ounces a day to give to a friend in exchange for yoga lessons. One donor asked me for a specific type of herb, with a precise brand and bottle size, to be purchased at Happy Day, our local, expertly stocked, but somewhat expensive health food store (and I was glad to oblige). Another donor asked if we would buy her an expensive electric pump (suggesting that if we paid for it, she would pump for both her child and ours). Of course the difference between gift and barter is somewhat heuristic, with expectations of further interaction significantly lowered under barter conditions that specify remuneration. But when milk is priced according to the principle of supply and demand and when money changes hands along with milk, there is no pretense of bartering, much less gifting. The milk becomes, in an anthropological sense, a commodity (see Kopytoff 1986).

As a commodity, milk has a monetary value. But how is the price established? Is some milk more expensive than others? If so, why? How might an economist analyze the market for milk? I was fascinated to read in Susan B. Draper's (1996) "Breast-Feeding as a Sustainable Resource System" that although breast milk is usually ignored in national resource inventories, it could significantly impact national portfolios, as well as national medical and environmental costs.

Institutions use an algebra of value to price their milk. Milk banks adhere to a hierarchy of neediness, but even insurance companies recognize that it costs less in the long run to provide NICU patients with expensive banked milk enhanced with fortifier than it is to allow them to consume cheap formula. So although shared milk is free, milk also already has a market value. It is routinely sold by milk banks and companies and at times commodified by private individuals. I would be surprised if more stringent legislation for this market is not on the horizon, but as is true for other areas of the law, legal guidelines regarding breast milk are poorly understood by the general public. Under what circumstances is it legal to buy and sell milk? Can sellers, website owners, or buyers be held responsible for trafficking in tainted, damaged, or adulterated milk? Given the significant amount of milk circulating, how might federal or state governments use tax codes to regulate sales?

As I mentioned in chapter two, milk is not included in the National Organ Transplant Act, which regulates the sale of organs, and many states exclude replenishable materials such as sperm or plasma from laws regulating the sale of bodily materials. Debates about whether we can or should sell bodily materials rarely center on breast milk. Laws in states that do regulate milk sales (California, New York, and Texas) pertain only to milk donated to a licensed milk bank, not to individual sellers participating in what David (2011) calls a "gray market."[4]

So under the current state and federal laws informal milk sellers may be liable only under limited circumstances, namely by engaging in fraudulent or negligent misrepresentation. Tort law could be brought to bear in cases of selling milk known to contain HIV or to be adulterated with other substances, but given the perishable nature of milk and the fact that most buyers have no way to test it upon receipt, it is unlikely that buyers would prevail in potential lawsuits (David 2011, 211).

In exploring how regulatory law might be used, Lori Andrews (cited in Waldeck 2002) notes that given the expected insolvency of providers of bodily materials, tort liability has little practical consequence; she suggests that criminal liability might be an effective means to ensure the quality of bodily materials offered in the marketplace. And in February 2010 a Tennessee lawmaker introduced a bill that would have made it a misdemeanor to sell human milk through informal channels such as the Internet, but the bill never made it out of committee review (David 2011, 165).

Why all the legal interest in sales of breast milk? An article provocatively titled "Bodies Double as Cash Machines with U.S. Income Lagging" (Stilwell 2013) reports that in all but two quarters since 2011, "hair," "eggs," or "kidney" have been among the top four autofill results for the Google search query "I want to sell my . . . ," according to Nicholas Colas, chief market strategist at New York–based ConvergEx Group, which provides brokerage and trading-related services for institutional investors. Kidney sales are illegal, but hair, semen, milk, and eggs can be sold, and in the context of neoliberal America people are looking for creative ways to make ends meet. Debating whether or not breast milk *should* be commodified is by now a moot point. We can still ask, What does it mean to describe the body as a cash machine? And what are the responses, meanings, and consequences to the push for body farming or industrialized, biocapitalistic milk commodification? What, if any, are the possibilities for a progressive politics within such a landscape?

Milk Matters

Is wet-nursing a form of body farming? With the considerable pressure on mothers to breastfeed and make a living (goals that are incompatible at times), a wet nurse revival might be in order. I have in fact noticed an uptick in the frequency of ads offering wet-nursing services in Georgia on sites like Only the Breast. Here is an example:

> Healthy, organic, clean, gluten free, mostly vegan, water from a spring. Wet nurse: No Adult Wet-nursing, No Pictures, No Videos, No Checks accepted, and No Scams. Donation to a BABY ONLY! If you do not have a needy baby and cannot pay via paypal then do not reply. I am a 25 year old mother of a 5 year old daughter and am expecting a baby in April 2015. My daughter nursed until she was four simply because I allowed her to self wean. My diet for the last four years has been organic, gf [gluten free], clean, and 90% vegan. I do eat eggs that come from our chickens that are feed [sic] organically in our back yard. I was looking for a nanny position but, then I thought becoming a wet nurse for another baby would be such a beautiful process. The value of breast milk is incredible but the actual breast nursing provides probiotics that aid in healthy digestion for life. If the situation is conducive I may be willing to relocate for the time your bundle of joy is nursing.[5]

So even as there are wet nurses looking for employment, the American public has yet to embrace wet-nursing, perhaps because of the idea that affection between baby and mother may be diminished by wet-nursing.[6] (Or maybe the cost is prohibitive: the annual salary requested for this "healthy, organic, clean, gluten free, mostly vegan, water from a spring" wet nurse was $97,000.) Perhaps the future is in farmed or even manufactured breast milk.

From our earliest evolutionary inception we have been tool-using cyborgs, organo-technological hybrids. If we compare the externalization of force through early choppers and scrapers with our ability to transform the global biome using fossil fuel technology and advanced genetic manipulation, we can see that the line between nature and culture is, and has always been, both ideological and dubious.

In fact *Wired* magazine has reported that an interdisciplinary team at the Counter Culture Labs (a DIY bio-lab) in Oakland, California, used mail-order DNA to trick yeast cells into producing a substance molecularly identical to cow's milk, a substance that they plan to turn into a kind of vegan cheese for people who do not want to consume animal products (Wohlsen 2015). The procedure can be used to synthesize milk from any mammal: the team is also planning to develop a version of what is known as Real Vegan Cheese that would be made with synthetic narwhal milk. And not surprisingly, human milk. The idea is that this "vegan" human cheese could be consumed by those with allergies to nonhuman dairy products. (The FDA, however, has placed a temporary kibosh on the human cheese experiment, citing concerns about auto-immune reactions). Author Marcus Wohlsen (2015) admits that vegan human cheese might not seem like a best-seller, but he notably avoids any discussion of human cheese as something perfectly consumable already (a point to which I return below).

This outlier science reflects an expansion of biotech interest in human breast milk that might one day challenge milk sharing, which until quite recently remained a relatively quiet practice. Transforming in real time from pressures originating both within and without, making it difficult to study and analyze but exciting to track, milk sharing is changing and becoming louder (and more visible). As I have depicted it, sharing by a counternetwork coalescing around a social-technological assemblage circulates milk along with knowledge and meanings attached to it. It is also within this counternetwork that milk comes to matter.

Matter is a special word. It can be used as a verb, as in something that matters; its transitive use means that something matters relationally, *to someone*. *Matter* can be used as a noun, to describe material, as in veg-etal or dark matter, as stuff. *Matter* can be made plural, as in matter(s): materials, or issues to consider. Matter has a perceptual aspect, where out of all the many, even infinite, possibilities, we specify attention to THIS or THAT set of things or ideas. We say, "We have several matters to cover today," to mean a group of issues, items significant or dear. Or the opposite, as in, "What is the matter? What is wrong? What is the prob-lem?" *To matter*, as a verb or as a noun, is *to appear* in some sense, to relate to, to become an object of perception, to affect.

In studies of material culture, matter is never a given but something that *emerges*. Some "thing" comes to matter, arrives as significant, because of circumstances, because of the relationships around it. We intend ourselves into the world through our interactions with matter. Matter, as *hui*, is a fundamental medium of knowing the world, relating to each other, and thinking about ourselves. This act of intending our-selves into and receiving the world, what we might call *living*, can be accomplished with milk or diamonds or cars or cities or even through what Timothy Morton (2013) has called hyperobjects, things like fossil fuels or the English language or other entities of such vast temporal and spatial dimension that they defeat traditional ideas about what a thing is in the first place. And crucially, a distinctly political semiotic question asks which matter counts, for whom, and how.

Matter can elide into a gerundlike form, *matter-ing*, that attracts and repels. It invites, and it orders (in both the categorical and imperative senses of the term) behaviors, relationships, sensations, ideas, values, and actions, of people, technologies, and organizations of every stripe. Matter-ing is implicated in the production of networks, counternetworks, or scenarios. Matter-ing, as the artist Joseph Beuys has shown us, shifts the world into focus in particular, and quite directed, ways.[7]

The avant-garde artist Guy Debord and the group Situationist International knew this. Their *situations* (which combined dadaist and sur-realist art to critique the triumph of commodity culture) matter-ed. As a practice, anthropology has a similar bent. Milk sharing also casts ques-tions into relief by enacting an alternative to the hegemonic world; sharers do this by refusing to snap to grid and by resisting the hyperob-ject of advanced neoliberal capitalism, with its profit motive, rational-ized social relationships, denial of the aleatory, and marketization of every aspect of life.

Matter is also implicated in infrastructures, delivering water or elec-tricity, for example, as well as for those less obviously but equally engaged in producing the starkly unequal arrangements of cultural subjects. This might be opaque matter, like milk or seeds, or wispy matters, such as identity or knowledge. And of course there are technological, economic, and political underpinnings that determine what and how things come to matter and, by the same token, how *what comes to matter* enables or frustrates citizenships, policies, or styles of resistance.

Scholars have considered matter-ing in their examinations of human-nonhuman relations and looked for ways that agency might be distrib-uted across social fields and material culture. I see the concept of distributed agency resembling the use of the term "matter" in astronomy, where it can be recognized by the effects exerted on other entities that may or not share its nature. For us terrestrials matter is exercised within a superlocal universe: the presence of a gun, or a green space, or a plaque, or a dripping breast, does things; it exerts itself.

So matter, like milk, is an event, is action oriented. It is a process. We can think of milk exerting an influence on other entities around it. Good anthropology has a history of calling out what matters, of matter-ing, by exploring the exercise of political power, the construction of hierarchies, the transformation of institutions, processes of subjectification, and interpretation of policy. Thinking about the frictions of matter as it moves through the world, pulled or repelled by other entities, casts light upon these questions by revealing how power is aimed at, shunted through, constituted or resisted by the experience of material objects, and vice versa. What are the crucial points of contact between the material and the political? How is matter enrolled in the execution of or resistance to social and moral regimes? Anthropologists try to figure out how political ideologies exerted through design, education, law, and management reproduce power structures or create opportunities for critique, if not dissent, in a variety of contexts. As I am presenting it, matter has a complicated ontological status, but just because something relates, acts, and interacts with other things in the world does not yet allow us to give it agency.

As I understand agency to work, that is to say, in cahoots with subjectivity if not intentionality, it seems very counterintuitive (given the worldview into which I have been deeply socialized and from which I am now writing) to characterize shoes or rocks or cords as agentive beings (even though at times it seems like, and I even behave as if, they are trying to trip me up) as is sometimes done in work that interrogates or collapses a subject-object dichotomy.[8]

It's unremarkable to back-engineer agency on the part of milk sharers: I assume they, like me, have subjectivities and that those subjectivities, like mine, include intentions (or at least what feels like intentionality) that seem to motivate various (apparently) goal-oriented actions. In contrast, when I think about a glass of milk, I do not immediately project an underlying subjectivity, although as an explorer I am more than happy to consider the possibility that my own worldview is just ideology, and

I admit to having ruined more than one family gathering by arguing with my brother about the consciousness of carrots, partly for sport, partly in seriousness.

Luckily the question of whether material objects have agency of the kind I usually believe humans might have is not one I need to answer right now. What is at stake here is a pragmatic rather than a theoretical question, because material culture like milk has real effects. It limits and/or encourages other entities (those with intention and those without) to have relationships or interactions with it. And in this interactive sense we might say that material culture acts in the world. This seems to be what Bruno Latour and other actor-network theory (ANT) scholars are keying into when they use the term "actant" or "agency."

In a fascinating critique of ANT Tim Ingold (2008) argues against the notion of symmetrically distributed agency, in which elements of an assemblage operate in relation to each other, none having more agency than another, by valuing instead the role of attention and responsiveness that accompany the developing nervous system in emergent life. He writes, "To attribute agency to objects that do not grow or develop that consequently embody no skill and whose movement is not therefore coupled to their perception, is ludicrous" (2008, 215). For the purpose of analyzing milk sharing, I find Ingold's critique, summarized by what he calls SPIDER (an acronym for skilled practice involves developmentally embodied responsiveness), useful for examining differently abled social agents: some spiders (social agents) have large powerful webs, while others are shy and tend to stay hidden; some spiders can and do kill and eat their mates, while others will attack and consume anything that moves.

In human society "skilled practice" (or power) is unevenly distributed. Within an anthropological context, discerning different kinds of power is essential to understanding both the reproduction and the disruption of the status quo. Sometimes this power is institutional; at other times it is physical, creative, intellectual, charismatic, or economic. Milk sharers wield all of these, with differing degrees of success, to get milk to matter.[9]

New Questions and Pressures

When I explained milk sharing to my own mother, she had questions. Having seen a news report about samples acquired via the Internet being cut with cow's milk, she said, "What are you trying to pull here anyway? This researcher proves that there is no telling what is in donated milk, so is it a really good idea to tell people how great it is and that they should go and get it?"[10]

I understood where she was coming from. I clarified that my intention is not necessarily to encourage people to seek donated milk but to describe how and what it means that parents already share.[11] I also explained that Keim's 2015 study collapses milk bought anonymously online with milk donated locally.[12] Nevertheless it is true that any milk could be contaminated or adulterated; not all milk is the same, which becomes apparent once we open questions about source, storage, and processing. We can begin to tease this out by considering the contours of distribution. And we must analyze shared, donated, and commodified milks separately and identify who has access to what.

My mother pointed out that although access to donated and commodified milk is shaped by race, class, and gender, people can generally buy and sell what they like as long as they have the means. So why, she wondered, if it can be adulterated or contaminated, wouldn't the state step in? The state could regulate it, tax it to pay for the oversight, and then make sure all of those who need it have it, and have it safely. Why not promote state control? These are perfectly reasonable questions, but for sharers any state control may be unwelcome for a variety of reasons.

For one thing the interests of stakeholders in milk distribution do not all coincide: individuals, milk banks, the state, and commercial entrepreneurs have different goals. People oppose the commodification of milk for a variety of reasons. It may be viewed as a sacred substance, profaned through commodification. Mothers may be willing to give it to a baby but will not sell to a company that plans to turn around and sell it at a profit. Others are completely at home buying and selling milk in any context.

Donors, donees, doulas, and milk bank personnel I spoke with were sensitive to the ways in which commodification and state regulation bring new questions and pressures to bear. I remember feeling unpleasantly suspicious when we received cold calls for milk sales. If I were truly desperate for cash and could sell my own milk, it might cross my mind to add water, formula, or cow's milk to the supply. With breast milk bringing up to three or more dollars an ounce, deception might make sense under certain circumstances: maybe I could get a higher price by fudging information about drug use, alcohol, and caffeine consumption, organic food intake, the age of my own baby, or the length of time frozen and type of freezer used, or other factors that might affect the quality or taste of the milk. These possibilities may not occur to everyone, but I would be surprised if no one considered them.

Similar to the way that sharers use the Internet to find donors or donees, people looking to buy or sell breast milk use Internet sites such as Craigslist or Only the Breast.[13] A recent Craigslist ad titled "Breast milk, not just for babies," bragged that "breast milk is one of the healthiest things you can drink, even for adults. Many star athletes drink it to boost their healthy calories and benefit from the antibodies. If you'd be interested in the . . . health benefits that breast milk has to offer then contact me and we can discuss. Just to clarify, I am happily married and not looking for anything sexual. I am looking to sell frozen breast milk to men or women who are interested in the health benefits." Interestingly this ad appears in the "strictly platonic" area of the personals section aimed at adults, not mothers and their babies.

Another Craigslist ad aimed at parents of infants states, "Pumped breast milk . . . $2.50 an ounce . . . have never smoked I don't drink. I don't used [sic] drugs of any kind. I have a healthy one month baby." It is impossible to say how successful these pitches were, and there are few Craigslist ads selling milk in my area (usually fewer than two per day). But OTB is extremely active, featuring thousands of postings; the home page says it all:

> Buy, sell or donate breast milk with our discreet classifieds system in a clean, safe and private way. Want to donate breast milk to a fellow mother? Considering selling or donating to a needy baby? Need natural breastmilk for your growing baby? Do you believe breastfeeding is best? Are you over producing and want to list your liquid gold for sale? Looking to make a few extra bucks while clearing out your freezer? Post a free ad and help babies get Only The Breast.[14]

OTB offers classified sections for donation and wet-nursing, but it is geared for sellers and buyers. Ads promoting sales are subdivided by baby age, discounted or bulk sales, milk produced by mothers with fat babies, fresh milk on demand, bank-certified and screened milk, local and fresh milk, milk produced by moms with special diets (vegan, gluten free, etc.), and moms willing to sell to men. Subdivisions of buyers mirror these categories, with additional ones for premature and sick babies. Most milk is priced between one and three dollars per ounce.

Like posts on donation websites, a typical seller's ad describes the mother's location along with details about diet, smoking and drinking habits, vitamin intake, reason for selling the milk, whether blood work is available, and how milk was procured ("I pump into sterilized bottles and immediately freeze the milk into freezer bags" and so forth). Sellers sometimes provide details about personal beliefs and practices not apparently related to milk production: This seller practices karate. That seller is Christian. This pediatric RN donor has more than three hundred ounces of frozen milk. OTB ads often contain photographs of the mother, the baby, or the freezer stash. Sellers may specify preferred buyers, as in, "I want to help a mom who doesn't have enough milk, or is unable to breastfeed." Another seller posts, "I am willing to sell to men." A typical ad reads like this:

> Very healthy new mother of a 1-month-old girl. I am pumping more breast milk than my little one can drink. She is exclusively breast fed, no bottles. I have been taking prenatal vitamins for over 2 years. I'm a nonsmoker, nondrinker, and I do not take any medication. I always pump my milk in sterilized bottles and freeze in 5oz breast milk freezer bags. My milk is really fresh as she is only 1 month old so I pump everyday all day. I only deal in frozen milk. I'm asking $2.00 per oz. You pay shipping and cooler/dry ice costs ($30–$50). No Adult Wet-nursing, No Pictures, No Videos, No Checks Accepted, and NO SCAMS! Pay Pal Payments ONLY!

In my community attitudes about commodification at times shifted depending on the recipient. Some mothers were willing to sell to bodybuilders or to adults who want to use breast milk in the course of erotic play. Warnings to parents and bodybuilders alike about buying milk refer to various studies by Keim (2013, 2015) and suggest people purchase it from banks (see Bakalar 2013). Insofar as the state has (re)discovered the benefits of milk for ensuring optimal outcomes and biopolitical governance, it has little tolerance for rhizomatic communities like a breast milk sharing counternetwork. Acting outside of easy surveillance and circulating a bodily substance coming to be seen as having greater and greater economic value, sharing and banking are not surprisingly attracting more federal interest. The U.S. Surgeon General's (2011) call to action on breastfeeding recommends a systematic review of the safety and health benefits of banked milk, the development of evidence-based guidelines for the use of milk, and establishment of federal guidelines for regulation and financial support of donor milk banks.

While administrators of Internet sharing sites welcome federal guidelines and resources for parents without access to banked milk, banks that are part of the Human Milk Banking Association of North America and acquire (free) milk from donors worry that sharing and for-profit companies (like Prolacta, Glycosyn, Jennewein Biotechnologie, Glycom, and Medolac) that pay for milk may be siphoning off valuable resources. In response HMBANA has turned to the persuasive power of concerns about ethics and safety, as seen in a press statement asserting support for unpaid donations: "relying on volunteer donors is the only ethical way to collect and distribute the human milk donations critically ill infants desperately need" (HMBANA 2014, 2). Proponents of donation also worry that greater commodification may result in a higher incidence of adulterated milk and to women "farming" their milk, possibly increasing output unsafely. An additional concern is that companies buying breast milk may coerce poor women into selling their milk instead of giving it to their own hungry babies.[15]

A Replenishable Source of Capital

The commodification of milk by both institutions and individuals is increasing.[16] Prolacta Bioscience, maker of Prolact+ H2MF, started paying mothers about $1 per ounce in 2014, processed an incredible 2.4 million ounces, and aimed to process 3.4 million in 2015 (as compared to the 3.5 million ounces handled by the combined efforts of all nonprofit HMBANA banks). Their fortifier, which provides extra calories, fat, and protein to babies, is manufactured in a 67,000-square-foot pharmaceutical-grade facility in Los Angeles that reportedly cost more than $18 million to build; with Prolacta pushing insurers to cover product costs (its product sold for about $180 an ounce in more than 150 national NICU units, with a total cost of approximately $10,000 per hospital stay per baby), there is a lot at stake. Prolacta pushes insurers and hospitals to pay by arguing that they will save money in the long term because research, in Prolacta-sponsored trials, suggests that fortifier wards off necrotizing enterocolitis (Lopez 2013; Pollack 2015).

Not surprisingly Prolacta has received more than $45 million in investments from life science venture capitalists who believe that breast milk, like blood plasma, can serve as a foundation for "valuable medical products"; Prolacta's CEO has explained that milk is "brimming with potential therapeutics, not only for babies but possibly for adults, to treat intestinal or infectious diseases, like the bowel ailment known as Crohn's disease" (quoted in Pollack 2015).

OTB cofounder Glenn Snow also saw gallons of white gold flowing through his site. He started his own (rather deceptively entitled) International Milk Bank to buy and process milk from his own site to sell to hospitals, explaining "it's a fascinating industry, and it's brand new" (quoted in Pollack 2015).

We are now witnessing the creation of new commodities from existing forms of life. Biocapitalism represents a fundamental shift in our understanding of boundaries between nature and culture and between human and nonhuman. This is the monetization of life, bodies, and body parts. When considering milk in this context, we would want to identify who is benefiting from its circulation, whether distribution is fair and equitable, what the relevant laws require of participants, how suppliers are being treated, and how issues of class are addressed in resource collection and distribution.[17]

To explore these questions the performance artist Miriam Simun staged *The Lady Cheese Shop est. 2011*. Having tracked the rise of artisanal foods at farmers' markets in New York City, she became interested in the politics of class, labor, and consumption. By making and serving cheese made from human milk, she engages her audience in a critical conversation about food and highlights politics surrounding the body.

"I tried to find a cheese maker to help me, but no one would touch this with a ten-foot pole! But then I found Heather Paxton's [2010, 2012] work. She is an anthropologist at MIT who works on artisanal cheese production and the role of bacteria, so I ran with her ideas," Simun explained. To use bioart to critique biotech, she produced different cheeses based on the diets of women from whom she procured milk. Her cheeses were blends: "I used cow or goat milk to augment the human milk because it does not coagulate on its own . . . the casein content in human milk is not as high in concentration," Simun explained. "I made a bleu cheese, for example, using a combination of human and cow milks, and a ricotta from a human and goat milk blend."

Simun's work targets the growing focus on, and concomitant pricing of, organic and artisanal foods, as well as what she calls "grand language" about hyperlocal and hypernatural foods (the same language, incidentally, used to create value in online posts to donate milk). She explains, "One thing I was interested in was the construction of *terroir* as 'an established character of a place.' I used this idea to reflect upon the obsession with local food in the urban environment: wild, the natural, the urban all coming together."

Food pairings at the *Lady Cheese Shop* opening were based on *terroir*, a term usually associated with fine wines, tea, or foie gras. She made a bleu cheese using milk from a mother living in Chelsea who liked apples, the farmers' market, and oatmeal cookies; the bleu was served with an oat cracker smeared with apple butter. The woman whose milk was used to make the ricotta cheese was Chinese, and she liked sweets; the ricotta was accompanied by black tea, orange cake, and ginger.

Tastings were free and public interest in the show was intense: "there was a line out the door, and [it got] a lot of varied reactions." To get a sense of what participants thought about the show, Simun offered comment cards to participants: "Some loved it and felt like it was adventurous, and wrote that I was dialing into eating as a next new thing. . . . Lactivists who are working on the normalization of breastfeeding, vocal critics of the fact that breastfeeding has to be hidden or the idea that babies should have their face covered when they are feeding, are fighting a perception that breastfeeding should be done in private and that it should be all hush-hush and at home. They were really appreciative of the concept, [suggesting that] it popularized the idea of accepting human milk." But not everyone, she explained, was a fan: "Some [people] were freaked out. . . . Adding value using terroir, a strategy that

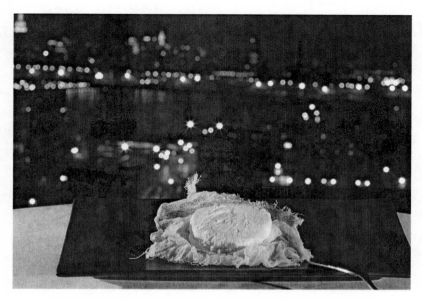

27. *Human Cheese, Urban Pasture.* Inkjet print on metallic paper. From
The Lady Cheese Shop, est. 2011. Courtesy of Miriam Simun.

creates the possibility for people to demonstrate an ability to discern,
to make ever finer distinctions between otherwise virtually identical
commodities, for human milk is just going too far."

A second dimension of the *Lady Cheese Shop* project addressed effort
and commodification. "For me," Simun said, "it is about the labor." Before
finding local donors, she bought milk on the Internet; she paid $2.50 an
ounce (plus a bit more for blood tests and shipping costs) to a seller in
Wisconsin (a state well known for its cheeses). This made sense because
selling sites like OTB offer highly territorialized milk—that is to say, the
milk is located in a particular place and attached to a particular person
who has a specific diet and lifestyle. Terroir is used, per Simun, to add
value, to create distinctions between hyperlocalized human milks. In
her work, breast milk cheese is offered as a quasi-artisanal product in
keeping with practices of social sorting within advanced commodity
capitalism of the kind Bourdieu (1984) outlines. The effect is to both
encourage and make strange the entire process.

But *Lady Cheese Shop* is really not that far out. Breast milk is found

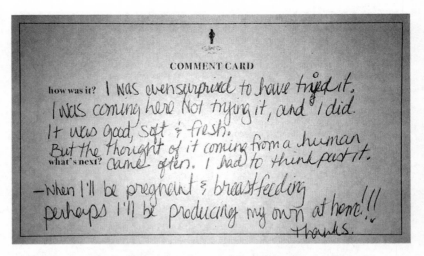

28. *Producing My Own at Home*. Audience comment card. From *The Lady Cheese Shop, est. 2011*. Courtesy of Miriam Simun.

(and contested) in recent culinary applications. The *Telegraph* (2008) has reported that a hullabaloo erupted when a major Swiss restaurateur posted ads asking for human milk, which would be used at Storchen, his restaurant at an exclusive resort in Winterthur. Hans Locher planned to offer stews and sauces made with human milk, which he (like Simun) said needs to be blended with whipped cream for consistency. His plans were foiled, however, by the Zurich food control laboratory because human milk is not on their list of approved species, such as sheep and cows.[18] Soon afterward New York chef Daniel Angerer of Klee Brasserie reported that his "phone was ringing off the hook" when it became known that he was cooking with his wife's breast milk, "so I prepared a little canapé of breast-milk cheese with figs and Hungarian pepper." Although some were too squeamish to try it, public feedback was generally positive. The response by the Department of Health was not: "the restaurant knows that cheese made from breast milk is not for public consumption, whether sold or given away" (quotes from Cartwright 2010).

Some entrepreneurs have been more successful than Locher and Angerer. Icecreamists, an ice cream shop in London, began selling a new flavor called Baby Gaga in 2011 (BBC News 2011). Baby Gaga is made with breast milk blended with Madagascan vanilla pods and lemon zest.

Perhaps its success can be explained by the fact that it is served in a martini glass with liquid nitrogen and rusk (and whiskey upon request) by a costumed waitress. (Could this be read as a more playful version of the Korova Milk Bar scene in Stanley Kubrick's dystopic *A Clockwork Orange*, in which "moloko plus," a drug-laced milk, is served from the nipples of furnishings shaped like naked women?)[19]

Decidedly less sexualized but similarly modern, milk distributed by banks and commercial businesses is also blended and standardized; it is deliberately *deterroirized*.[20] Commercial milk products are uniform and cannot be traced to any one mother. Milk banks also aim for a standardized product because they operate within a universe of hospitals, insurance companies, and customers who demand a standardized, deterritorialized product.

But even standardized milk needs to be placed within a landscape of interpretations. Jane Khatib-Chahidi (1992), for example, shows that milk kinship, which ritually achieves all kinds of objectives (from making peace between tribes, to consolidating clan unity, to preventing marriages, to creating clients) may operate beyond a nursing woman's own interests. Ideas about milk's ability to produce kinship may result in an aversion to consuming banked milk in the United States, where banks may mix together milk from three or more anonymous donors. How would one know who and where their new kin are?

We might imagine a future in which the captains of biocapitalism construct milk as a valuable national resource and call on ecological qualities such as climate, humidity, wind, temperature, or dew, which give varieties of paté or Darjeeling tea their various price points.[21] One might imagine branded milks that do not identify individual moms but do highlight diet (lactose free), exercise (yoga), environment (country living), mental health, or intelligence (high IQ) in recalling age-old ideologies about ideal characteristics of wet nurses. Branded milks could not only be stamped with approval by the state, perhaps by the FDA, but would easily slide into established commodity consumer practices.

This step would mark the elision of milk into a full-fledged market commodity, like branded chocolates or wines, that Simun's *Lady Cheese Shop* implicitly questions. Who, under current economic conditions, could be surprised to see branded milks sold at various price points that would allow consumers to enact class- or other identity-based performances similar to those in place for other baby goods such as strollers, diaper cream, and shampoo? "Home-made" milk may even come to be derided as a cozy and nostalgic but lesser foodstuff, an unfortunate alternative for those who cannot afford biocapitalized milks. With biotechnologists already hacking yeast cells to produce synthetic mammalian milk, the need for women to make any milk at all could be eradicated. One might even imagine specially engineered "supermilks" becoming the nutrition of choice for babies and adults alike.

By way of considering this hypothetical, I found it interesting that some of Simun's audience had responded, as she explained, to *Lady Cheese Shop* "by calling it 'cannibalistic' [on the response cards]." Simun then suggested that this response is "of course, . . . highly irrational, but in saying this, people are reflecting a struggle, and they were searching for the right words to describe their feelings." This struggle, really against the abject, has also been taken up in popular films. For example, Richard Fleischer's film *Soylent Green*, released in 1973, is a whodunit set in a dystopian future (in the year 2022) in which jobs and food are scarce; most people live on wafers said to contain ocean nutrients. Detectives working to solve the murder of an elite with access to "real food" discover that the wafers are made from the only available form of protein left: human bodies. They urge everyone to recognize that "Soylent Green is people!"

More recently, and more in keeping with the construction of human milk as white gold, the giddy fourth installment in the postapocalyptic Mad Max film series shows human breast milk on par with gas and water as a vital, coveted substance to be farmed from women and for adult consumption. Most characters in George Miller's 2015 film *Mad Max: Fury Road* are experiencing what Giorgio Agamben calls "bare life," as bodies that may (or may not) be called up by those in power to be used as soldiers, as "blood bags," or milk makers to uphold, or to expand, the status quo. While *Fury Road* is a caricature, the implied critique of a biopolitical state that regards people as resources for maintaining the state rather than as subjects with inalienable, natural rights is clear. In bare life whatever agency people have left is exerted by and at the site of the body, their very life being the only card they have left to play.

Critics of commodified milk worry about the consequences of farming that we see sketched in *Fury Road*. But the shock value of milk as it appears in *Fury Road* is gained in part from Miller's gamble that his audience would view this portrayal as beyond the pale. Ironically milk's abject status, in which drinking it is viewed as "cannibalistic," may be what protects it from moving into large-scale branded industrial production.

Adventures with Others

Sharers often mentioned the commodified body in interviews. Jodi told me that she had "even nursed two friends' babies, and they nursed mine. It is just not a big deal even though some people think that it is weird. And why? I mean think about it: milk is for babies!" She went on to discuss breastfeeding a baby as sacred labor:

> I mean, I am not a vegan, but I am intrigued by it, and I feel like it is bizarre that we drink cow's milk or milk from other animals. But then, we think human milk is weird! My experience as a lactating mammal has given me a new perspective on this whole thing, about what is weird, or what is gross. I mean pumping is not a big deal and I was happy to do it, but it is not that it is so great either. It can be uncomfortable or even hurt. It makes me think of cow's milk as being more of a big deal than I ever thought it was before. Put it this way: we were at a petting farm, and there was a dairy guy there doing an exhibit about his cows and the process of milking and everything, and so, the cow was hooked up to a pump. And my friend and I were like, "Oh my god, what if that were us, hooked up with a bunch of people ogling at us!" It is just not respectful. It's terrible. And it's not respecting the miracle that milk is. I think few people really stop to consider it like that.

It is hard to imagine people like Jodi, who was both a donor and a donee, accepting industrial milk commodification. But in response to growing pressures HM4HB Facebook administrators remind users that "our site is for donation and needs only. Selling milk on our page is not permitted. We encourage our community to ask questions publicly and call out those who are found to be selling. Thank you for your cooperation. Ps. Bartering is a form of commerce and trading milk for other items is prohibited. Asking to replace milk bags is acceptable" (HM4HB 2015).

The larger power dynamics were not lost on Issa, our doula. She explained that her concerns were with "profit-motivated meddling with women's work. Because, of course, now the 'institution' is moving to regulate breast milk. So who can donate milk and how is under more scrutiny, and really, right now we are at a crux, a cross in the road. This is a shifting time, because we see big business on the horizon. It may be that donors will become part of that business, with government regulation, and then milk will come only from donors who are underwritten by those entities. This is what happened with midwifery."

She explained how midwifery became institutionalized and medicalized in ways that have been both helpful and harmful, but very much controlled by men: "Now having said that, all around here there are 'underground midwives.' One in particular is absolutely terrific, but she is not licensed, not legal, but you can be sure that people come from miles around to go to her. So I am guessing that donation may also become more controversial, that is to say less 'authorized,' and end up going somewhat underground. Right now is the time to look at this shift."

Being someone who thinks a great deal about access and knowledge, from the rational and scientific to the local and intuitive, Issa is sensitive to changes in women's motivations to sell or gift: "You can see how if breast milk starts to be a more saleable item, people might feel like they should sell their milk. And maybe that's not so great. . . . As a donee, you would have to have really good insight if that starts to happen. Being a commodity can change it, but I see that as more of a continuum. It may be that milk that is sold can still work in a personal relationship, but yeah, you definitely have to consider a lot of other things when we go from donation to sale."

Part of the conversation we were having about commodification was also a dance around sociality and payment. We had hired Issa to provide what might have been, in another time or place, provided by family members—mothers, sisters, or aunts. Issa was my doula, and believe me, we were more than happy to pay her to help us because I was totally clueless about how to take care of a new baby, and although unbelievably excited, I was also kind of terrified. She came to help me again with our second child, but over the four years we have now known each other she has visited with us, we have been to her home, and we run into each other around town. As we discussed the commodification of breast milk, there seemed to be an unspoken comparison—what about a doula?

I was happy that we could talk about these very questions: Does paying for something always mean that business interests rather than personal ones reign? To what extent is human feeling diminished if payment is involved? Perhaps relationships enabled by commodified versus donated breast milk could work on a continuum, some participating in it strictly for the money while others do it for the emotional satisfaction or, for some, a bit of both. After all, both donors and donees I spoke with described a range of sharing relationships: some were deeply personal while others had little sociality.

An adventure is an enterprise with no known outcome or destination. On the adventurous nature of his Light Pavilion in the Raffles City complex in China, the architect Lebbeus Woods (2011) wrote, "Whether it will be a pleasant or unpleasant experience; exciting or dull; uplifting or merely frightening; inspiring or depressing; worthwhile or a waste of time, is not determined in advance by the fulfillment of our familiar expectations, because we can have none, never having encountered such a space before. We shall simply have to go into the space and pass through it, perhaps more than once."

I often felt like this myself, wondering where milk sharing would take us, and I learned to see it as an adventure in living, partly thanks to my reading of Woods, a topic that I will take up in the next and final chapter.

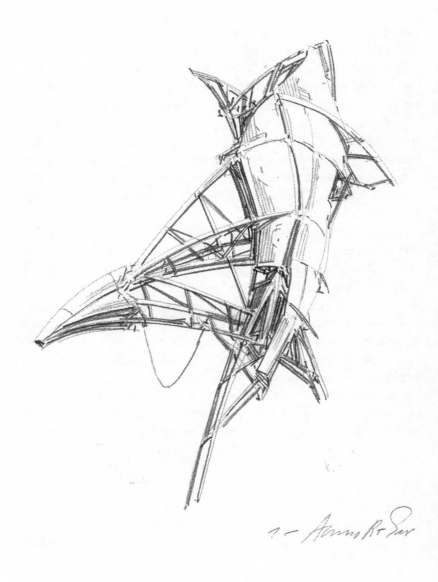

29. Lebbeus Woods, architect, American (1940–2012), *Untitled (Aerial Paris)*,
1989. Graphite on paper, 9½ × 12½ inches. Previously unpublished. © Estate of
Lebbeus Woods.

6   Free Space

> Now there is no choice but to invent something new, which
> nevertheless must begin with the damaged old, a new that neither
> mimics what has been lost nor forgets the losing, a new that begins
> today, in the moment of loss's most acute self-reflection.
>
> LEBBEUS WOODS, *Radical Reconstruction*

Milk sharers from different walks of life become entwined in an emergent, negotiated community shot through with technology, ideas, and
materiality. This community is powered by an explicit, and rather self-
conscious, "us-them" critique of official policy. While sharing breast milk
does reproduce some of the values it seeks to resist, for example, ideas
about gender, this practice remains a transformational "site," with small
acts by many people having the potential to make a big difference. Milk
sharing and the ideologies that power it infuse a larger cultural context.
As Law (2009) has pointed out, patterned practices, once they are established, can reproduce themselves, spreading realities from site to site
in forms that hold their shape. As a patterned socio-techno-material
practice that is reproducing itself, milk sharing becomes ever more
mainstream each day but still promises an array of undiscovered critical
possibilities and outcomes.

The local sharing community functions as grassroots action. Families
respond to authoritative medical discourse and commercial advertising
with a refusal to abdicate. They have created an anarchistic heterarchy,
one in which not only breast milk but also ideas about children, parenting, capitalism, and society are exchanged. This adventure in living
together well is a mode of dissent. And just as the shift toward decentralized forms of organizing, networking, education, and exchange using

social media may ensure the sustainability of the experimental Free University, the Occupy movement, Greece's barter economy, and other sociopolitical explorations, the fact that the population sharing milk is shifting and nebulous enhances the counternetworks' ability to avoid, and even resist, surveillance or regulation from above.[1]

Milk sharing is based on want and surplus, but participants also describe how a desire for self-sufficiency; a longing to avoid commercialism associated with babies; a mistrust of the pharmaceutical, medical, and food industries and governmental bodies; and a commitment to support local communities drive participation. But what are the broader implications of sharing? How might an examination of sharing help us to develop other radical imaginations? Where can we look for alternative visions?

Architecture and Anthropology

> It is crucial that we invent strategies for seeing the familiar differently. If we rely solely on seeing it in familiar ways, we will only be able to reenact what we have already done and confirm what we already know.
>
> LEBBEUS WOODS, *Slow Manifesto*

Because art and anthropology have the power to unsettle knowledge-producing practices (Buckley 2016; Maskovsky 2013b), anthropologists and artists have worked together to make the world visible in particular ways and to envision new futures. As an art form aimed at designing the world we inhabit, architecture in particular has much to share with anthropologists. But how might we incorporate the work of collectives like Superstudio and Ant Farm or that of individuals like Michael Benedikt, Victor Papanek, Juhani Pallasmaa, and Lebbeus Woods into ethnography or theory?[2] How might these architectures shape an anthropology of the future?

The future is only and always a construct that animates the present, helping us to picture utopian or critical design solutions to human problems—political, ecological, social, or material. Considering the future can encourage us to envision living in new ways. Architects, like urban planners, community leaders, and even Wall Street Occupiers, are tasked with placing themselves into an imagined future when developing strategies for meaningful intervention, all the while knowing that they may fail. But what futures are at play and how might the contours of these futures shape contemporary action or theory? Future play in art and design can operate as meaningful critique, as has been demonstrated in the work of Victor Papanek and Buckminster Fuller, both of whom have inspired lasting transformations.

The value of visionary work is not always immediately apparent. Papanek (1971), an erstwhile ethnographer, was once ostracized for using recycled materials and promoting design solutions for poor people but is now celebrated as a great father of sustainability studies and design. Fuller made it his mission to enrich human life through energy-efficient designs that were also trenchant critiques of wasteful consumption. His iconic geodesic domes and use of what he called "design science" have been replicated all over the world. The architect Lebbeus Woods advanced a similarly radical aesthetic that can enrich the anthropological imagination.

I came to link design with anthropological futurity from an admittedly oblique angle, one that suggests a methodology for looking at future-oriented activities. As a project, this is an adventure, in the sense that it has an uncertain outcome, but the act of exploring, of trying, of looking to exceptional thinkers in parallel fields has in itself always strengthened the anthropological effort.

So besides recognizing Woods as an exceptional artist and thinker, I have had my eye on his work for some time as a key to understanding milk sharing in the context of a speculative anthropology of the future. It occurred to me to do this because of the long-standing dialogue between art and anthropology, from French ethnology's relationship with 1930s surrealism, the rise of phenomenologically inspired ways of looking and theorizing the body in the 1970s (Merleau-Ponty 1964), the avant-garde inspired experiments of the "writing culture" debates in the 1980s (Clifford 1988; Marcus and Fischer 1986), and most recently what Hal Foster has called the "ethnographic turn" within the arts themselves (Strohm 2012; Foster 1996). Most borrowings move from anthropology to art, but as Arnd Schneider and Christopher Wright (2006, 2010) argue, art practices can invigorate our scholarship by suggesting new ways of seeing. What's more, this attention to the aesthetic realm should not simply be taken as an appendix to knowledge making, as several anthropologists have recently pointed out.

Rupert Cox, Christopher Wright, and Andrew Irving (2016) argue that insofar as different sensory experiences are implicated in knowledge making, we need to develop creative forms of representation that diverge from correspondence theories of truth. Ingold (2013) also calls for a recalibrated relationship between art and anthropology: while there is a long and venerable lineage of the anthropological study of art, it has, not unlike the discipline of art history, taken art as an object, symptomatically, as an index of cultural or political configurations. That's a dead end. Why not activate an anthropology *with* art, where both are taken as practices that reawaken the senses to allow knowledge to grow from the inside of being (Ingold 2013, 8)? Could art, Ingold writes, not be regarded as form of anthropology, albeit "written" in nonverbal media? Here I would suggest that anthropology can itself be a form of art, not in the sense that it might contain nonverbal expressions like sketches, poems, or musical compositions or that it is expressed through visual media like film or photographs, but that anthropology *is* art in the best sense of art, as a technique.

There are many definitions of art, some more interesting than others. I recently attended a talk at a museum in which the visiting artist, Anne Ferrer, announced that art should be pretty and make her feel happy. The remark elicited applause. This is not what I mean when I say that anthropology can be art. What I mean is that anthropology, like art as described by Viktor Shklovsky, can have a dehabitualizing effect; it can make the familiar strange. In "Art as Technique" (1917) Shklovsky wrote that "art exists so that one may recover the sensation of life; it exists to make one feel things, to make the stone stony. The purpose of art is to impart the sensation of things as they are perceived and not as they are known. The technique of art is to make objects 'unfamiliar,' to make forms difficult, to increase the difficulty and length of perception because the process of perception is an aesthetic end in itself and must be prolonged. . . . Art removes objects from the automatism of perception" (quoted in Kolocotroni, Goldman, and Taxidou 1999, 19).

An excellent example of anthropological work with a dehabitualizing effect, what Shklovsky called *ostranenie* (**остранение**), is Horace Miner's classic about the "Nacirema" (1956). Here Miner presents American society through the lens of a purportedly ethnocentric other so that Americans can see themselves anew. Like good art, successful anthropology makes the familiar strange and the strange familiar. The experience of *ostranenie* has a lasting impact on our perception, on our insertion in the world. Successful anthropology should not only be defined by representational accuracy or the production of elegant theory; it should stick to you. It transforms your mind. It adheres to the bottom of your feet, changing the way you feel and think as you walk through the world. It makes you recover the sensation of life, of *being* alive.

True story: this happened when I was reading Paul Stoller's *Stranger in the Village of the Sick* (2005), a book about different ways of *being in the world*, about remaining open to fieldwork, and about illness and sorcery. My husband and I were taking a friend to a nearby U.S. military base. I knew from visiting there previously that everyone in the car would need to show a government-issued ID to enter the base, but I had forgotten to bring my purse. I silently commanded the soldiers not to see me sitting in the backseat: "I am invisible to you." As expected, we were stopped at the gate. The guards opened the doors and checked the documents of the passengers in the front seat. Then one of the guards opened the back door. I sat as still as a stone. He did not see me (or if he did, he pretended not to). I felt like the sorcerers' magic was working through me. I felt an extraordinary sense of possibility and of being alive.

Fieldwork in Niger changed Paul Stoller. His book changed me, altering how I understand and move in the world. Same with Michele Stephen's *A'aisa's Gifts* (1995) and Vincent Crapanzano's *Tuhami* (1980). I could list many other books, some ethnographic, others theoretical, that have had a profound effect on me. These anthropologies are, I submit, works of art, not the happy, pretty kind but the kind that dehabitualizes. For me, good anthropology, like good art, is an *experience*.

Art in all media—painting, literature, sculpture, and architecture—can do this. I am especially interested in architecture, as the discipline shares with anthropology a concern for exploring creative processes that give rise to the environments we inhabit and to the ways we perceive them (Ingold 2013, 10). Both are invested in changing the world for the better and have benefited from at times painful, internal critiques about reflexivity, representational practices, and colonial histories.

The rise of the architectural critique developed in the 1960s when architects, in an attempt to redress problems associated with modernism, began integrating social context into theory.[3] This critique resulted in the rise of community design, user-centered design, sustainable design, and so forth, which depart in significant ways from traditional paradigms.[4] Today many well-known practitioners engage in activities that are both defamiliarizing and imaginative, producing designs that provide innovative, pragmatic solutions to pressing problems.[5] In this sense architecture (like anthropology) shows itself to have both diagnostic and therapeutic tendencies. Work by Lebbeus Woods certainly falls within this domain. (I am sure you are by now wondering what happened to breast milk. Please stay tuned. I will get back to that.)

Living by a Different Set of Rules

> Architecture and war are not incompatible. Architecture is war.
> War is architecture. I am at war with my time, with history,
> with all authority that resides in fixed and frightened forms.
>
> LEBBEUS WOODS, *War and Architecture* 1993

Lebbeus Woods, a master of architectural *ostranenie*, was born in 1940 and died in 2012, not long after he wrote his last blog entry, entitled "GOODBYE [sort of]," in which he presciently announced that his days of regular posting were over.[6] He had studied engineering at Purdue University and architecture at the University of Illinois before working for Eero Saarinen Associates from 1964 to 1968 and then teaching at Cooper Union (and many other schools) until the end of his life. Obituary headlines described him as unconventional, visionary, and futuristic.[7] And although Woods's work was rarely realized, was indeed unrealizable, he stated, "I'm not interested in living in a fantasy world. . . . All my work is still meant to evoke real architectural spaces. But what interests me is what the world would be like if we were free of conventional limits. Maybe I can show what could happen if we lived by a different set of rules" (quoted in Yardley 2012).

A desire to suggest what these different rules might be seemed to animate much of Woods's work. Explicitly concerned with issues of justice, freedom, and human creativity, he was critical of the role of capital interests in producing violence of all kinds: structural, military, economic, bureaucratic, and symbolic.

Reflecting upon conflict and crisis as forces within which architectural forms take shape, Woods (1993) wrote, "Social justice is not an issue of masses, but of individuals. If the mass is satisfied with its salutes, but an individual suffers, can there be justice, in human terms? To answer 'yes' is to justify oppression, for there are always people willing to lose themselves in a mass at the expense of some person who is not willing to do so. To construct a just society, it is precisely this lone person who must first receive justice. Call this person the inhabitant. Call this person yourself." It is the job of the architect to not only be that person but also to design for that person. Much of Woods's work is, then, in dialogue with architecture itself, an exploration of ethical practice.

Woods spent a great deal of time designing for landscapes that had suffered war, economic siege, and natural disaster and for the "people of crisis" living in places like Berlin, Sarajevo, Cuba, San Francisco, and even New York. Woods viewed human life as sets of small movements that can have a cumulative effect, with urban sites serving as vectors of activity that could become infused into the larger political matrix. The potential for cultural change is thus located in agents operating within highly designed spaces, usually created by architects who are charged with upholding institutions of authority rather than liberating inhabitants in any real way.

Woods's liberation aesthetic is particular and recognizable, especially once you see examples of his illustrations for novels and poetry.[8] His work, featured in a retrospective at the San Francisco MOMA and at the Drawing Center in New York, is hand drawn and collagelike in a world in which architectural renderings are usually accomplished using computer programs such as Revit or AutoCAD and then peppered with premade digital "scalies" (images of people that give scale, populate, and suggest functionality in computer-rendered images of buildings or cityscapes). Such software snaps projects to grid, by which I mean they become legible in terms of hegemonic political, economic, and even cultural ideologies and underpin the increasing homogeneity of global design.

Most scalies are well behaved and attractive. They have a tendency to be clearly gendered and of the middle and upper classes. They are used, for example, to confer an emotional or even aesthetic appeal to developers and other viewing publics. Rarely does one encounter scalies that appear in any way that might be considered ambiguous, critical, or ugly. You can be sure that there are few women scalies with visibly leaking breasts or engaged in breastfeeding, except perhaps in art projects that are explicitly using scalies as a raw material or that are addressing the ideological use of scalies.

In this vein the artist James Bridle (2013) places scalies within the category of what he calls "render ghosts," or "people who live inside our imaginations, in the liminal space between the present and the future, the real and the virtual, the physical and the digital . . . in space which exists only in the virtual spaces of 3D computer rendering software, projected onto billboards, left to rot and torn down when the actual future arrives; never quite as glossy or as perfect as our renderings of it would like it to be, or have prepared us for." Render ghosts are simultaneously ideological and utopian; they foster the status quo as imagined by those who are designing it.

Participants in Rob Walker's (2015) Hypothetical Development Organization subvert the hegemonic use of scalies in all kinds of ways: for example, a scantily clad scalie solicits johns outside a Loitering Center, and a paramilitary-style guard rides a Segway around a fortresslike Reading Room. This work shows how scalies operate as visual rhetoric, tied to seducing viewers into embracing a renderer's pitch rather than simply depicting actual use. It is too bad that Walker's plan to create a set of "off" scalies, such as panhandlers, obnoxious tourists, or menacing police officers, was never realized, as it would provide a toolkit for students to engage in architecture as critique.

I have seen few scalies in Woods's work, and when they do appear they are hand-drawn figures that reflect his overall project; scalies shopping or kayaking (apparently a popular trope in contemporary rendered backgrounds that imply trendy sustainability, "green" architecture, and an engagement with nature) have no place here. Were you to examine his work, you would find that neither prefab scalies nor digital software alone could accommodate Woods's imagination.

In his *War and Architecture* (1993), *Radical Reconstruction* (1997), and elsewhere Woods designs alternative realities. While most architects operate on the assumption of stability, he embraces change and the uncertain path of the human condition. He offers provocations to problems caused by political, structural, and natural violence and calls for energized engagement. For Woods architecture is "an instrument for the invention of, 'in Marcuse's words, new modes of existence with new modes of reason and freedom,'" instead of a link in the chain of command whose most important task is to design "spaces with 'functions' that are actually instructions to people as to how they must behave at a particular place and time" (Woods 1997, 22). We can look to the horizon but should refrain from programming future behavior.

In keeping with the idea of design for change Woods draws fascinating philosophical connections between notions of meaning and value under various political, scientific, and artistic regimes. Among his most fruitful is the observation that just as chaotic motion and self-referentiality—anathema to respectable science less than a century ago—have been incorporated into traditional logic systems and are even yielding practical results, there is no reason why the paradoxical space of uncertainty cannot also be dealt with "logically" within architecture (Woods 1997, 26). This celebration of uncertainty is related to another line of inquiry in which Woods, following Nietzsche, identifies the role of the poetic in evoking and resolving the paradoxical, without losing the creative potential that lies therein (22). In engaging not just technological innovations, such as computer-aided design, but also new conditions engendered by crisis and then by life in a postcrisis society, cultural activity can work not only as a mirror but also as a transformational lens through which we understand ourselves anew. Through making the familiar strange and the strange familiar, we have a chance to live in a different and, we hope, better way.

Woods's embrace of open-ended change and the (sometimes violent) energies that drive it as the essence of existence results in designs that draw on a set of provocative conceptual tools. Some of his tools are based on metaphors of the self-healing body, for example, *scab*, *tissue*, and *scar*. These can all be integrated into an anthropological lens, but I find the notion of free space to be the most useful.

Free Space

> Are we ready to live fearlessly in the present—accepting a
> future governed by probability—and to hone our minds and
> bodies to a degree of poise and agility that history has not
> known before? Or will we deny the imperatives of these
> understandings and sink back into the illusory comforts of
> mere history?
>
> LEBBEUS WOODS, *OneFiveFour*

One of the most provocative sites of uncertainty is Woods's "free space,"
introduced in his 1990 Berlin Free-Zone project (Woods 1991). In contrast to modernist "universal space" (which is actually a kind of disguised
multifunctional space), *free space* has no function, or "program," identified in advance. It only suggests a set of potentials for occupation aris-
ing from material conditions. In the Berlin project the material conditions
were a kind of hidden city, with unlimited, free access to the communications and networking equipment usually reserved for government or
commercial use. In free space inhabitants are unfettered by the conventions of behavior usually enforced by these institutions.

In the design, free spaces are like special interstices discovered by
chance or only by those who are looking for them. For those who make
the choice, free spaces offer a *terra nova*, a new ground of experience,
new modes of reason and freedom, and an instrument of critical transformation. What is gained is not necessarily an answer but rather an
articulation of the creative potential of paradox and the poetic. And in
order to participate, Woods argues, the practice of architecture must
itself be reconstructed, just as the architecture required by the changed
conditions of living must be invented anew.

This work can provide a scaffold for both an analysis of the present
and an anthropology of the future. One way we can do this is to look at
how we are already inhabiting free spaces, spaces that, as evoked by
Fernando Coronil (2011, 235) in his thinking on the future of Latin America, "appear to oscillate between the malleable landscape of utopian
imaginaries and the immutable ground of recalcitrant histories."

This would mean seeking out postcrisis landscapes, be they political,
social, structural, or natural, in which we find collaborative interactions

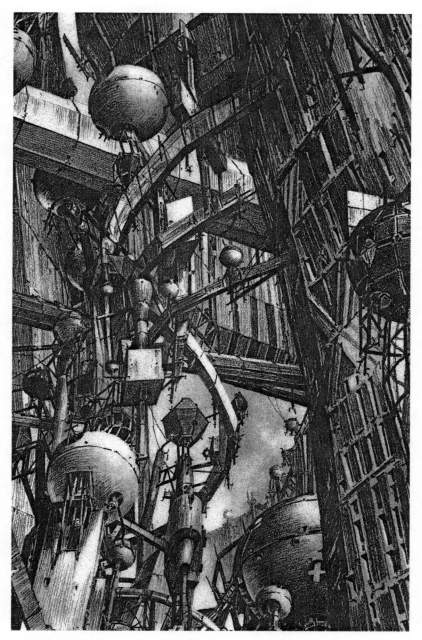

30. Lebbeus Woods, architect, American (1940–2012), *City of Fire*. From *Four Cities*, 1981. Graphite on board, 6 × 11 inches. © Estate of Lebbeus Woods.

taking place under the radar of the state or outside the gaze of authoritative institutions, which are both critical and seeking to enact an alternative. Analyzing what is happening in these real free spaces, how they shape and are shaped by relations of power, specifically with regard to questions of race, kinship, commodification, human-animal relationships, climate change, and so forth, will provide lessons both methodological and theoretical. By examining participation in extant free spaces we may find new ways to mobilize knowledge and to sketch workable models for future research, representation, and organization (see Maskovsky 2013a).

One such free space for participation is the subject of this book: breast milk sharing. This almost-hidden counternetwork invigorates a community of erstwhile strangers who share a critique of food, medical, and pharmaceutical industries through an Internet- and technology-enabled exchange system that circulates information and milk and in some cases produces kinship. A refreshing example of relationship building, breast milk sharing exists parallel to, and perhaps because of, commodity capitalism. It is both a critique of and an experimental solution to problems posed by contemporary parenting.

What I find intriguing about this free space is the formation of what Woods, recalling Crumley (1995) and McCulloch (1945), calls a "heterarchy": a spontaneous, lateral network of people responding to an evolving situation, here represented by the profit motive as applied to the body and to childcare. As the breast milk sharing free space has become more visible between 2010 and 2016 (through news reports, newspaper articles, and Internet chatter), there is greater pressure for conformity to the larger society, to commodification, with more donees setting price points for milk rather than offering a relationship.

As breast milk sharing becomes better known, and thus available, the critical edge of this practice will be challenged. There is a sweet spot between the visible and the invisible, in which large numbers of participants creatively negotiate alternative relationships and operate parallel to hegemonic formations. But even if it is short-lived, I suspect that milk sharing will have long-term empowering effects on participants.

Here the architectural model provides a lens for the study of "people of crisis." Woods's free-space framework allows anthropologists to systematically identify and compare small-scale experiments in living and community making, as well as experiments in attempts to find local, workable, organizational responses to encroaching political, structural, and natural crises of a larger order. Some of these experiments will be successful, some will be nasty, and some will last longer than others, but all will operate in dialogue with the larger status quo, casting that status quo's critical points into relief. These are, however, hit-and-run solutions, constantly in danger of being absorbed by the maelstrom of capital and crisis and therefore inherently ephemeral.

Milk sharing is an experimental form of living together in free space and is thus under threat from ambient cultural environments, in this case capitalism and its ideologies of risk and total motherhood. Free spaces may ultimately provide only a brief respite but, when occupied, may enhance our ability to imagine, enact, and refine alternatives to a capitalism that not only sequesters knowledge about the rudiments of human life and health but that is actively destroying the very environment upon which human life depends.

I don't think this short-livedness would have bothered Woods, a person for whom equilibrium would have meant death: life, *real life*, is always emergent, responsive, and in flux. It requires taking a leap into the unknown. It requires not knowing the outcome in advance. It requires trusting each other. This valorization of the unknown is an affront to Enlightenment mandates to know and shows us Woods the maverick. I was gratified but not surprised to read Eric Owen Moss reporting that "'outside-the-box thinking has become a cliché used in advertising, corporate strategy and politics, but Woods took it to another level. There's another box, and he's outside it. He's outside all the boxes.'"[9] But as innovative as he was, we will eventually need free spaces beyond even those he imagined. Woods viewed his own work as pointing to a horizon beyond which no one could see. What does the milk horizon look like? Hacked yeast cells, milk farming, and branding will surely continue to challenge community sharing.

Sites like Only the Breast and companies like Prolacta do provide some revenue that many women need, but they also undermine the critical discussion encouraging and encouraged by milk sharing. There

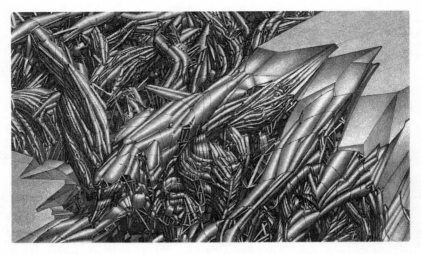

31. Lebbeus Woods, architect, American (1940–2012), *NEW TISSUE Landscape*, 1993. Graphite and colored pencil on board, 12 × 19⅞ inches. © Estate of Lebbeus Woods.

is something else happening in the daily thickening and thinning of this counternetwork, however. Milk sharing is powered by a politics of pragmatics, guided by a desire to meet specific goals, not to generate theory. In this sense sharing can look serendipitous, even idiosyncratic, at times. As a responsive, "live" practice, participants respond to each other as people trusted to be responsible for one other. In this sense breast milk sharing is a refusal, a resistance to, a rebuff to the demand to abdicate competency woven into contemporary regimes of governance. Sharers reserve the right to trust their own instincts; to identify, evaluate, and respond to risk; and to make decisions by and for themselves with unknown outcomes (see Goodman and Goodman 1960). As these competencies are increasingly given over to the state, to corporations, and to authoritative institutional others, one starts to wonder, What is the point? What does it mean to be *alive*? Where is the adventure? Where is the element of choice and open-endedness essential to the construction of an ethics? One way to *be alive* is to be radically embedded in a community of people whose fates are linked. And really, that's everyone.

An anthropology deliberately engaged with fugitive activities like milk sharing will be in a better position to appreciate how experimental practices and how people squatting in spaces designed for maintaining the status quo, showcasing hierarchy, and entrenching the values of capitalism might be embedded in the everyday.[10] By living a different present, these erstwhile squatters make imagining a different future seem possible.

Notes

1. Milk Moves

1. In a meditation on his own field books Michael Taussig (2011, 13) explores how "drawings come across as fragments that are suggestive of a world beyond, a world that does not have to be explicitly recorded and is in fact all the more 'complete' because it cannot be completed."
2. See excellent contemporary artwork by Lynn Randolph, Jess Dobkin, and Miriam Simun.
3. Artistic renderings of the Lactation of Saint Bernard may be found at the website WTF Art History, accessed November 20, 2015, http://wtfarthistory .com/.
4. "Founded in 1949 at Yale University, the Human Relations Area Files, Inc. (HRAF) is an internationally recognized organization in the field of cultural anthropology. HRAF's mission is to encourage and facilitate the cross-cultural study of human culture, society, and behavior in the past and present. HRAF produces two online databases: eHRAF World Cultures and eHRAF Archaeology, and other resources for teaching and research." HRAF website, accessed November 20, 2016, http://hraf.yale.edu/.
5. All figures in this paragraph and the next are from the American Academy of Pediatrics 2011 policy statement, "Breastfeeding and the Use of Human Milk," accessed July 12, 2015, http://pediatrics.aappublications.org /content/129/3/e827.full#sec-30.
6. See the entry by Kimberly Seals Allers (2013) in the *Motherlode* blog of NYTimes.com, where issues such as whether or not the AAP logo belongs on formula gift bags are debated.
7. La Leche League International, "History," accessed May 10, 2016, http:// www.llli.org/lllihistory.html.
8. Regardless of studies on contaminants, work policy, or gender politics, the idea that "breast milk is best" was well established by 2005 thanks to the combined efforts of AAP, LLL, the WHO, the CDC, and the FDA. According to the 2013 CDC Breastfeeding Report Card, rates of breastfeeding continue

to increase across the United States, with about 70 percent of all American mothers initiating breastfeeding and about 35 percent of infants receiving breast milk at six months (Centers for Disease Control 2013). There are regional variations: only 68.2 percent of women in Georgia ever breast-feed their babies, with 31.8 percent still breastfeeding at six months (6.2 percent exclusively). Only 12.9 percent still breastfeed at one year.

9. Providing a detailed account of the history of wet-nursing is outside the scope of this project, but see works by Apple (1987), Golden (1996), and Fildes (1987).

10. Elia Chepaitis (1985) writes in her doctoral dissertation that early and mid-Victorian adults consumed staggering amounts of opium and that administering opium to children was commonplace. In some areas opium feeding was nearly ubiquitous, although it was controversial in some circles. Engels and Marx mentioned child doping, and parliamentarians and medical men publicized the recklessness with which opiates were dispensed to infants. An Addiction Research Unit report (2001) from the University at Buffalo states, "Mrs. Winslow's Soothing Syrup was an indispensable aid to mothers and child-care workers. Containing one grain (65 mg) of morphine per fluid ounce, it effectively quieted restless infants and small children. It probably also helped mothers relax after a hard day's work. The company used various media to promote their product, including recipe books, calendars, and trade cards such as the one shown here from 1887 (A calendar is on the reverse side)."

11. That artificial feeding was used in ancient times is evidenced by the discovery of vessels in all shapes and sizes made from wood, ceramics, and cow horns and dating back thousands of years (Stevens, Patrick, and Pickler 2009). Stevens, Patrick, and Pickler show that between the sixteenth and eighteenth centuries mothers used Hugh Smith's "bubby pot" and pap boats (a milk and bread mixture) to supplement feedings. But these instruments were hard to clean, and so, combined with poor milk storage and sterilization, artificial feeding led to many deaths. A refined, more hygienic feeding bottle became available during the Industrial Revolution; by 1896 an open-ended, boat-shaped bottle had been developed in England. The development of better feeding technologies and a decline in society's acceptance of wet-nursing led to an increased use of alternative milk sources.

12. For details see the HMBANA website, accessed March 23, 2015, https://www.hmbana.org/.

13. The HMBANA website, https://www.hmbana.org/, explains each step of milk processing and provides a series of photos connoting scientific methodology, hygiene, and exactitude. Donated milks are pasteurized

according to the Holder technique (heating milk to 144.5 degrees Fahrenheit and holding there for thirty minutes, which decreases bacterial load but can also negatively impact nutritional value) and then mixed together.

14. The HM4HB website, accessed March 25, 2015, is https://www.facebook .com/hm4hb/info?tab=page_info.

15. The MilkShare website, accessed May 20, 2016, is http://milkshare .birthingforlife.com/.

16. The Only the Breast website, accessed May 20, 2016, is http://www .onlythebreast.com/.

17. The OTB website, http://www.onlythebreast.com/, explains the home pasteurization process: "Slowly heat the milk to 145 degrees Fahrenheit, stirring occasionally. If you are not using a double boiler, stir frequently to avoid scalding the milk. Hold the temperature at 145 F for exactly thirty minutes. You may need to increase and decrease the heat to keep the temperature constant. Remove the pot of milk from the heat and place it in a sink or large bowl filled with ice water. Stir constantly until the temperature drops to 40 F. Store pasteurized milk in the refrigerator."

18. From the International Milk Bank website, accessed April 29, 2015, http:// www.internationalmilkbank.com/contact/investors/.

19. There are many approaches to anthropological work on material culture (e.g., Falls 2008, 2014, 2015; Ingold 2013; Gottdeiner 1995; Hicks and Beaudry 2010; Law 2009; Meyers 2002; Prown 2001; Rotenberg 2014; Banerjee and Miller 2008).

20. Gold is weighed by the troy ounce (31.10 grams), which is the equivalent of 1.09714286 avoirdupois ounces (28.329 grams). Avoirdupois ounces can be used to measure everyday things like milk.

21. A feeling of discomfort, if not offense, with breastfeeding and the accouterments of milk among onlookers was echoed in a recent article in the *New York Times* parenting blog *Motherlode*. A working mother wrote in asking for advice because her office mate complained to the human resources department when she spotted a breast pump peeking out of a bag. The office mate "wants to not have to see the black bag because it grosses her out" (Belkin 2011).

22. For a fascinating collection of work describing how the meanings of goods are transformed as they pass through various state and/or cultural regimes, see the contributions to Schendel and Abraham's (2005) edited volume.

3. Breast Milk Is Best

1. See also works by Crumley and Marquardt (1987) and by Bondarenko, Grinin, and Korotayev (2002).

2. The finding in *Obergefell v. Hodges* required states to license marriage between two people of the same sex and to recognize a marriage between two people of the same sex when their marriage was lawfully licensed and performed in another state. See the Supreme Court blog, accessed October 15, 2015, http://www.scotusblog.com/case-files/cases/obergefell-v-hodges/.
3. These figures are based on data from the 2010 census analyzed by the Williams Institute and cited in "State Policy Profile—Georgia," Movement Advancement Project (MAP) website, accessed April 21, 2015, http://www .lgbtmap.org/equality_maps/profile_state/11.

4. Lactivism

1. A rendering of the nearby galaxy NGC6744 was taken with the Wide Field Imager on the MPG/ESO 2.2-meter telescope at La Silla, Chile. The large spiral galaxy is similar to the Milky Way, making this image look like a picture postcard of our own galaxy sent from extragalactic space. The picture was created from exposures taken through four different filters that passed blue, yellow-green, and red light, as well as the glow coming from hydrogen gas. Wikipedia, accessed June 13, 2015, https://commons .wikimedia.org/wiki/File:Wide_Field_Imager_view_of_a_Milky_Way _look-alike_NGC_6744.jpg.
2. For a deeper engagement with the many meanings of milk, see the discussion of Peircian type and tokens in the introduction to this book.
3. Agency is the ability of a person to act. In anthropological terms agency is often set up in a dialectical relationship with structure, one in which social facts—histories, policies, laws, practices, values, and norms—shape (or even define) the parameters of experience. The structure-agency debate revolves around the extent to which people refract or are determined by (or "written by") structures versus having the capacity to exert themselves. Work by poststructuralists such as Pierre Bourdieu (1984) attempted to reconcile the terms of the debate by recognizing subjects' varying abilities to strategically respond to circumstances that precede them in what is known as "practice theory." Practice theory is useful because it helps to explain the deeply conservative but emergent nature of both society and culture.
4. This suit was still under litigation at the time of writing (December 2015). ACLU, accessed May 11, 2015, https://www.aclu.org/cases/bockoras-v -saint-gobain-verallia-north-america.
5. See also "Pumped Up," NBC News, accessed May 11, 2015, http://usnews .nbcnews.com/_news/2014/01/10/22257760-pumped-up-breastfeeding -mothers-fight-for-rights-at-work?lite.

6. Section 4207 of the Affordable Care Act requires employers with fifty or more employees to provide reasonable break time and a private, nonbathroom space for nursing mothers to express breast milk during working hours for up to one year after the child's birth. The new requirements became effective when the ACA was signed into law on March 23, 2010. The current law applies only to nonexempt employees in jobs that are covered by the overtime provisions of the Fair Labor Standards Act (FLSA). Twenty-four states, Puerto Rico, and the District of Columbia also have policies supporting breastfeeding in the workplace. As of this writing, advocates are working to extend the reasonable break time allowance to exempt employees (salaried employees) and to expand the Civil Rights Act of 1964 to protect breastfeeding women from being fired or discriminated against in the workplace. For more information see "Break Time for Nursing Mothers," Wage and Hour Division, U.S. Department of Labor, http://www.dol.gov/whd/nursingmothers/. See also "Federal Support for Breastfeeding," AAP, accessed June 15, 2015, https://www2.aap.org/breastfeeding/files/pdf/FederalSupportforBreastfeedingResource.pdf.
7. Perhaps our squeamishness about sharing is due to, as Amber suggested, an "oversexualization of the breast combined with invasive formula marketing; we think we can filter it all out but it is the ads and everything else, and [sterile] formula is still a powerful norm."
8. See the overview of social movements by Edelman (2001).
9. The infrastructure has been replicated all across the United States and abroad such that once people have a basic understanding of how milk sharing works, they can access milk elsewhere. Our family took advantage of this replication when we traveled across the country, and we also received milk from donors passing through our home area. When vacationing in northern California, we used the HM4HB Facebook page to find Emily, a donor from Los Angeles who was also there for work. She was pumping while away from her own baby but did not want to throw the milk away; she provided us with fresh (not frozen) milk over a three-day period. Others told me of similar experiences, even in international travel.
10. Affect theory can run though a hip-hop aesthetic: Rich Homie Quan's "Type of Way" was released on August 22, 2013. It is the second single from his *Still Goin In: Reloaded* mixtape. Addressing the boyfriend of the girl he's seeing, Quan uses the phrase "some type of way" to describe a range of complex emotions—from jealousy to sexual attraction. For commentary, full lyrics, and video see "Type of Way," Genius.com, accessed June 1, 2016, http://genius.com/Rich-homie-quan-type-of-way-lyrics.

11. In 2014 the United Arab Emirates passed a law requiring mothers to breastfeed children for two years. Critics of the law point out that some mothers may not be able to breastfeed, that the new law could generate court cases by fathers against mothers who do not comply, and that it places an undue burden on mothers who are working or who choose not to breastfeed (Graham-Harrison 2014).

12. The 2012 declaration was obtained from the World Breastfeeding Conference website, accessed September 19, 2015, http://www.bpni.org /report/declaration-wbc2012.pdf.

5. Economic Matters

1. See interviews in the work by Jodorowsky (2009). I would also highly recommend Jodorowsky's many films (e.g., *El Topo, Santa sangre or Endless Poetry*), comics (e.g., *L'Incal*, with the French illustrator Moebius), and writings (e.g., his *Psychomagic* or *Way of the Tarot*). Frank Pavich's documentary *Jodorowsky's Dune* (2013) is an instructive introduction to the artist and the man.

2. Extended ethnographic research focused on the way a single commodity is interpreted by a community of consumers is rare, perhaps because of the difficulty of locating and interviewing people. And, although participants in my research for *White Gold* do not constitute a commodity community per se, they did participate in networked sharing of a single "good" that is increasingly becoming commodified. See the work of Radin (2001).

3. See Jane Guyer's new translation of Mauss's *The Gift*. Mauss ([1925] 2016, 197), Guyer argues, was writing out of an urgent need to find inspiration from other parts of the world, that Europeans might learn "to confront one another without massacring each other." Indeed I am detailing how the sharing of milk suggests new ways of being together.

4. California Health & Safety Code §§1647–48 (2010); N.Y. Comp. Codes Rules & Regs. 10 §§52.9.1–9.8 (2010); N.Y. Public Health Law §2505 (2010); 25 Texas Admin. Code §227.1 (2010); Texas Health & Safety Code Ann. §161.071 (2009).

5. Advertisement text from Only the Breast, accessed July 12, 2015, http://www.onlythebreast.com/breast-milk-classifieds/show-ad/44368 /healthy-organic-clean-gluten-free-mostly-vegan/pine-lakedecatur -30072/georgia/usa/wet-nurse-america/.

6. These same ideas were advanced by the seventeenth-century French obstetrician Jacques Guillemeau (1612).

7. For an introduction to both the work and the artist Joseph Beuys see the books by Beuys and Harlan (2004) and by Mesch and Michely (2007). I

would also recommend performance documentation. *Joseph Beuys – How to Explain Pictures to a Dead Hare* (located online at goo.gl/hCgY6z) is an excellent introduction to Beuys at work.

8. See Robert Rotenberg's (2014) extremely useful discussion of agency. He writes that agency is a quality of human beings that refers to the socioculturally mediated capacity to act, ordinarily understood as intentional and based on an agenda (36). Here someone acts, intending a certain result, and expects for others to understand it because they are similarly habituated. Of course both language and material culture are polysemic—they can contain both explicit and implicit meanings that modify, amplify, augment or even contradict one's intentions—but still, they can operate prosthetically.

9. Milk does do things, but it does things because of the way people are positioned to put, move, use, and interpret milk in the world. In his commitment to analyze language aside from its referential capabilities Austin (1962) shows how words do things, but nowhere does he say that words have agency. His book title is *How to Do Things with Words*, not "How Words Do Things," or "What Words Do"; in *How to Do Things with Words* someone enunciates words to some interpreter in a context. An agent is doing something by using words. The words do not do anything in and of themselves, or by themselves. In order for words to do anything they have to be noticed; they have to *matter*.

What words, or a string of words, can have are consequences. They cement or break apart relationships, create obligations or expectations, and mark or manage social hierarchies. Sometimes the consequences exceed the intentions of the speaker, while at other times they fall short. Words can be misunderstood, accidentally or on purpose. But however they come across they are understood by a community of users habituated to an interpretive regime. That is to say, interpretation is contextual and cultural. These interdigitated aspects of language—consequence, congruence, and habituation—help us to examine a semiotic dimension of material culture. As a semiotic vehicle, milk carries meanings, reflects an intention, operates as a prop in a performance of gender or parenthood or capitalism, or indexes a desire or value system, as can the act of giving, selling, or receiving milk. The interpretive regimes of sellers and donors overlap but are not congruent. Are they mutually constitutive? Will one eventually prevail over all? Clearly these questions are shot through with issues of power, agency, and habituation.

10. Keim et al.'s (2015) study found 10 of 102 anonymously purchased Internet samples with bovine DNA concentrations high enough to rule out

minor contamination, suggesting that a cow's milk product was added. Drinking cow's milk could cause problems for those with lactose intolerance or an allergy.

11. Admittedly, very few parents are involved in milk sharing. Nonetheless, casting hidden practices into relief is one of the most important outcomes of the anthropological project.

12. Keim's (2013) team purchased breast milk anonymously online, without requesting any information about the donor, without making personal contact, and without discussing the purpose of the milk (all actions that people seeking milk for a baby would likely take). In other words communication by the research team was incongruent with the kinds of requests usually made by real parents (see Stuebe, Gribble, and Palmquist 2014). This may have affected the care with which milk was prepared and shipped. On the other hand the milk that Keim's team tested from a milk bank did not show contamination. And although to my knowledge no baby has been sickened by donated milk, it is true that donated milk can be adulterated or contaminated, accidentally or on purpose, in ways that might be avoided in milk bank or commercial milk products because of their testing and product controls.

13. See Only the Breast, accessed March 15, 2015, http://www.onlythebreast .com.

14. Only the Breast, accessed October 20, 2014, http://www.onlythebreast .com/.

15. A compensation scheme with Brazilian donors in the 1940s was ended when it became clear that mothers' own infants were not being fed (Keim et al. 2015).

16. Paying for institutional facilities and staff, donor testing, processing, shipping, marketing, and so forth requires a good deal of money. But compared to the cost of medical or surgical management in a NICU unit for even one case of necrotizing enterocolitis or short bowel syndrome, these expenses are nominal. One study estimated savings to the California health care system of eleven dollars for every dollar spent on donor milk as a result of reduced medical interventions (HM4HB 2015).

17. Relevant work on new tissue economies can be found in the work of Waldby and Mitchell (2006).

18. See details on meals cooked with human milk in the *Telegraph* (2008).

19. The 1971 film *A Clockwork Orange* was Stanley Kubrick's adaptation from the 1962 novel of the same name by Anthony Burgess.

20. Against *deterroirized*, the more familiar anthropological term would be "deterritorialized."

21. See works by Besky (2013) and DeSoucey (2016) for analyses of the relationship between terroir, global consumer markets, and value.

6. *Free Space*

1. See the works by Maharawal (2013), Juris (2012), Berger, Funke, and Wolfson (2011), and Alderman (2015).
2. See representative works such as those by Benedikt (1987), Papanek (1971), Pallasmaa (2012), and Woods (1989).
3. For details see the work of Hays (1984), which views architecture as both cultural activity and critique.
4. From what I can tell, setting up the "program" (an architects' plan for what users are supposed to do inside of a design) remains an important aspect of training students. Its existence is rarely questioned.
5. *Volume* magazine, for example, explores architectural responses to the emerging challenges of new urbanity. For example, Rem Koolhaas, Todd Reisz, Michaal Gergawi, Bimal Mendis, and Tabitha Decker (2010) do this in a profile of six cities of the Persian Gulf region, from the air, from the ground, as design, historically, and architecturally, in the midst of financial crisis. Also see the article by Varughese (2013).
6. Woods's (2012) blog entry "GOODBYE, sort of" and many others have been published in an edited collection, *Slow Manifesto* (Woods 2015). The blog is a window into Woods's thought about the relationship between architecture, education, politics, and dissent. The entire blog is archived at https://lebbeuswoods.wordpress.com/.
7. Obituaries for Lebbeus Woods appeared in major newspapers, as well as in architectural blogs and journals.
8. For examples, see Woods's illustrations in works by Clarke (1983) and Bensen (1980).
9. An interview with Moss about Woods appeared in an article by Yardley (2012). See also the article by Trounson and Ng (2012).
10. "If you believe in the world you precipitate events, however inconspicuous, that elude control, you engender new space-times, however small their surface or volume" (Deleuze 1995, 176). Being, thus, is doing.

References

ACLU. 2013. "Bockoras v. Saint Gobain Verallia North America." ACLU, last modified November 6. https://www.aclu.org/cases/bockoras-v-saint -gobain-verallia-north-america?redirect=cases/reproductive-freedom /bockoras-v-saint-gobain-verallia-north-america.

Addiction Research Unit. 2001. "Before Prohibition: Images from the Prepro-hibition Era When Many Psychotropic Substances Were Legally Available in America and Europe." Retrieved from https://wings.buffalo.edu/aru /preprohibition.htm.

Akre, James E., Karleen D. Gribble, and Maureen Minchin. 2011. "Milk Sharing: From Private Practice to Public Pursuit." *International Breastfeed-ing Journal* 6 (8): 1–3.

Alberti, L. B. (1438) 1751. *Vita anonymae.* In *Rerum Italicarum Scriptores XXV,* edited by L. Mehus. Milan.

Alderman, Liz. 2015. "Trading Meat for Tires as Bartering Economy Grows in Greece." *New York Times,* September 21, International Business. http:// nyti.ms/1iIaIt5.

Alinsky, Saul D. 1989. *Rules for Radicals: A Practical Primer for Realistic Radicals.* New York: Vintage.

Allers, Kimberly Seals. 2013. "Does the A.A.P. Logo Belong on Formula Gift Bags?". *Motherlode,* (blog entry) NYTimes.com, last modified December 19. http://parenting.blogs.nytimes.com/2013/12/19/does-the-a-a-p-logo -belong-on-formula-gift-bags/?_r=0.

Altorki, Soraya. 1980. "Milk Kinship in Arab Society: An Unexplored Problem in the Ethnography of Marriage." *Ethnology* 19 (2): 233–44.

Anand, Nikhil. 2011. "PRESSURE: The PoliTechnics of Water Supply in Mumbai." *Cultural Anthropology* 26 (4): 542–64.

Anand, Nikhil, Johnathan Bach, Julia Elyachar, and Daniel Mains. 2012. "Infrastructure: Commentary." Curated Collections, Cultural Anthropol-ogy website, November 26. https://culanth.org/curated_collections/11

-infrastructure/discussions/6-infrastructure-commentary-from-nikhil
-anand-johnathan-bach-julia-elyachar-and-daniel-mains.

Anderson, Leon. 2006. "Analytic Ethnography." *Journal of Contemporary Ethnography* 35 (5): 373–95.

Apple, Rima D. 1987. *Mothers and Medicine: A Social History of Infant Feeding, 1890–1950*. Madison: University of Wisconsin Press.

Arnold, Jeanne E., Anthony P. Graesch, Enzo Ragazzini, and Elinor Ochs. 2012. *Life at Home in the Twenty-First Century*. Santa Fe: University of New Mexico Press.

Asad, Talal, ed. 1973. *Anthropology and the Colonial Encounter*. New York: Humanities Press.

Atkin, Albert. 2013. "Peirce's Theory of Signs." In *The Stanford Encyclopedia of Philosophy*, edited by Edward N. Zalta. Stanford CA: Metaphysics Research Lab, Center for the Study of Language and Information, Stanford University. http://plato.stanford.edu/archives/sum2013/entries/peirce -semiotics.

Austin, J. L. 1962. *How to Do Things with Words*. Cambridge MA: Harvard University Press.

Avishai, Orit. 2011. "Managing the Lactating Body: The Breastfeeding Project in the Age of Anxiety." In *Infant Feeding Practices: A Cross-Cultural Perspective*, edited by Pranee Liamputtong, 23–38. New York: Springer.

Bakalar, Nicholas. 2013. "Breast Milk Donated or Sold Online Is Often Tainted." *New York Times*, October 21, online edition. http://nyti.ms /18i84Fd.

Ball, O. 2010. "Breastmilk Is a Human Right." *Breastfeed Review* 18 (3): 9–19.

Banerjee, Mukulika, and Daniel Miller. 2008. *The Sari*. London: Berg.

Barclay, Barry. 1990. *Our Own Image*. Auckland: Longman Paul.

Barlow, Kathleen. 2010. "Sharing Food, Sharing Values: Mothering and Empathy in Murik Society." *Ethos* 38 (4): 339–53.

Barlow, Kathleen, and Bambi L. Chapin. 2010. "The Practice of Mothering: An Introduction." *Ethos* 38 (4): 324–38.

Barston, Suzanne. 2012. *Bottled Up: How the Way We Feed Babies Has Come to Define Motherhood, and Why It Shouldn't*. Berkeley: University of California Press.

Barthes, Roland. 1973. *The Pleasure of the Text*. Paris: Éditions du Seuil.

Bayat, Asef. 2000. "From 'Dangerous Classes' to 'Quiet Rebels': Politics of the Global Subaltern in the Global South." *International Sociology* 15 (3): 533–37. doi: 0.1177/026858000015003005.

———. 2010. *Life as Politics: How Ordinary People Change the Middle East*. Amsterdam: Amsterdam University Press.

BBC News. 2011. "Breast Milk Ice Cream Goes on Sale in Covent Garden."
February 24. http://www.bbc.com/news/uk-england-london-12569011.

Beers, Robin, and Jan Yeager. 2012. "Open Source Family: Implications for
Remaking and Renewing Notions of Family." *Ethnographic Praxis in
Industry Conference Proceedings* (1):368–70.

Belkin, Lisa. 2011. "Offended by an Office Breast Pump" (blog entry). *Motherlode*, NYTimes.com, last modified July 7. http://parenting.blogs.nytimes
.com/2011/07/07/offended-by-an-office-breast-pump/?_r=0.

Benedikt, Michael. 1987. *For an Architecture of Reality*. New York: Lumen
Books.

Bensen, Robert. 1980. *In the Dream Museum—Red Herring Chapbook No. 6*.
Urbana-Champaign IL: Swamp Press.

Benyshek, Daniel. 2010. "Eating the Placenta: How Do the Nutritional and
Hormonal Profiles of Unprepared Human Placental Tissue Compare with
Processed Human Placenta Capsules?" American Anthropological
Association Annual Conference, November 17–21, New Orleans.

Berger, Dan, Peter Funke, and Todd Wolfson. 2011. "Communications
Networks, Movements and the Neoliberal City: The Media Mobilizing
Project in Philadelphia." *Transforming Anthropology* 19 (2): 187–201.

Berle, J. O., and O. Spigset. 2011. "Antidepressant Use during Breastfeeding."
Current Women's Health Review 7:28–34.

Besky, Sarah. 2013. *The Darjeeling Distinction: Labor and Justice on Fair-Trade
Tea Plantations in India*. Berkeley: University of California Press.

Beuys, Joseph, and Volker Harlan. 2004. *What Is Art? Conversations with
Joseph Beuys*. West Sussex UK: Clairview Books.

Blum, Linda. 1999. *At The Breast: Ideologies of Breastfeeding and Motherhood
in the Contemporary United States*. Boston: Beacon Press.

Boccaccio, G. (1351) 2003. *The Decameron*. Translated by G. H. McWilliam.
2nd ed. New York: Penguin.

Bondarenko, Dmitri M., Leonid Grinin, and Andrey Korotayev. 2002. "Alternative Pathways of Social Evolution." *Social Evolution & History* 1 (1):
54–79.

Boswell-Penc, Maia. 2006. *Tainted Milk: Breastmilk, Feminisms, and the
Politics of Environmental Degradation*. Albany: State University of New
York Press.

Bourdieu, Pierre. 1984. *Distinction: A Social Critique of the Judgement of Taste*.
Cambridge MA: Harvard University Press.

Bridle, James. 2013. "The Render Ghosts" (blog entry). *Electronic Voice
Phenomena*, November 14. http://www.electronicvoicephenomena.net
/index.php/the-render-ghosts-james-bridle/.

Brooks, Elizabeth. 2012. *Legal and Ethical Issues for the IBCLC*. Burlington MA: Jones & Bartlett.

Brown, Michael. 1996. "On Resisting Resistance." *American Anthropologist* 98 (4): 729–35.

Buchan, William. 1769. *Domestic Medicine, or, A Treatise on the Prevention and Cure of Diseases*. Edinburgh: Balfour, Auld, Smellie.

Buckley, L. 2016. "Ethnography at Its Edges: Bringing in Contemporary Art." *American Ethnologist* 43 (4): 745–51.

Buzard, James. 2003. "On Auto-Ethnographic Authority." *Yale Journal of Criticism* 16 (1): 61–91.

Bynum, Caroline Walker. 1987. *Holy Feast and Holy Fast: The Religious Significance of Food to Medieval Women*. Berkeley: University of California Press.

Carroll, Katherine. 2012. "Introducing Donor Human Milk to the NICU: Lessons for Australia." *Breastfeeding Review: The Professional Publication of the Australian Breastfeeding Association* 20 (3): 19–26.

———. 2015a. "Breast Milk Donation as Care Work." In *Ethnographies of Breastfeeding: Cultural Contexts and Confrontations*, edited by Tanya Cassidy and Abdullahi El Tom, 173–86. New York: Bloomsbury Press.

———. 2015b. "The Milk of Human Kinship: Donated Breast Milk in Neonatal Intensive Care." In *Critical Kinship Studies*, edited by C. Kroløkke, L. Myong, S. W. Adrian, and T. Tjørnhøj-Thomsen, 15–33. London: Rowman and Littlefield International.

Carter, Pam. 1995. *Feminism, Breasts and Breast-Feeding*. New York: St. Martin's Press.

Cartwright, Lachlan. 2010. "Wife's Baby Milk in Chef's Cheese Recipe." *New York Post*, March 9. http://nypost.com/2010/03/09/wifes-baby-milk-in-chefs-cheese-recipe/.

Cassidy, Tanya. 2012. "'Milky Matches': Globalization, Maternal Trust, and 'Lactivist' Online Networking." *Journal of the Motherhood Initiative* (Special Issue on Motherhood and Activism) 3 (2): 226–40.

———. 2014. "Mothers, Milk, and Money: Maternal Corporeal Generosity, Sociological Social Psychological Trust, and Value in Human Milk Exchange." *Journal of the Motherhood Initiative* (Special Issue on Motherhood and Economics) 3 (1): 96–111.

Cattelino, Jessica. 2010. "The Double Bind of American Indian Need-Based Sovereignty." *Cultural Anthropology* 25:235–62.

Centers for Disease Control. 2013. *Breastfeeding Report Card for the United States 2013*. Atlanta GA: Centers for Disease Control and Prevention, Division of Nutrition, Physical Activity, and Obesity. Accessed November

20, 2016, at http://www.cdc.gov/breastfeeding/pdf/2013Breastfeeding ReportCard.pdf.

Chang, Heewon. 2008. *Autoethnography as Method*. Walnut Creek CA: Left Coast Press.

Chepaitis, Elia Vallone. 1985. "The Opium of the Children: Domestic Opium and Infant Drugging in Early Victorian England." PhD diss., University of Connecticut.

Cheyney, Melissa. 2010. "The Tree of Life as Postpartum Medicine: Placento-phagy and the US Homebirth Movement." American Anthropological Association Annual Conference, November 17–21, New Orleans.

Clarke, Arthur C. 1983. *The Sentinel*. New York: Berkeley Books.

Clifford, James. 1988. *The Predicament of Culture: Twentieth-Century Ethnog-raphy, Literature, and Art*. Cambridge MA: Harvard University Press.

Colburn-Smith, Cate, and Andrea Serrette. 2007. *The Milk Memos: How Real Moms Learned to Mix Business with Babies—and How You Can, Too*. New York: Tarcher.

Cole, Juan. 2010. "Saudi Clerics Promote Kinship by Sharing Breast Milk" (blog entry). *Informed Comment: Thoughts on the Middle East, History and Religion*, June 9. http://www.juancole.com/2010/06/saudi-clerics -promote-kinship-by-sharing-breast-milk.html.

Contreras, Randol. 2012. *The Stickup Kids: Race, Drugs, Violence, and the American Dream*. Berkeley: University of California Press.

Coronil, Fernando. 2011. "The Future in Question: History and Utopia in Latin America (1998–2010)." In *Business as Usual: The Roots of the Global Financial Meltdown*, edited by Craig Calhoun, 231–92. New York: New York University Press.

Cox, Rupert, Chris Wright, and Andrew Irving. 2016. *Beyond Text? Critical Practices and Sensory Anthropology*. Manchester UK: Manchester Univer-sity Press.

Crapanzano, Vincent. 1980. *Tuhami, Portrait of a Moroccan*. Chicago: University of Chicago Press.

Craven, Christa. 2005. "Claiming Respectable American Motherhood: Homebirth Mothers, Medical Officials, and the State." *Medical Anthropol-ogy Quarterly* 19 (2): 194–215.

Crumley, Carole. 1995. "Heterarchy and the Analysis of Complex Societies." *Archeological Papers of the American Anthropological Association* 6 (1–5). doi:0.1525/ap3a.1995.6.1.1.

Crumley, Carole, and William H. Marquardt. 1987. "Regional Dynamics in Burgundy." In *Regional Dynamics: Burgundian Landscapes in Historical*

Perspective, edited by Carole L. Crumley and William H. Marquardt, 609–23. New York: Academic Press.

David, Stephanie Dawson. 2011. "Legal Commentary on the Internet Sale of Human Milk." *Public Health Report* 126 (2): 165–66.

Davis, Allison, Burleigh Gardner, and Mary Gardner. (1941) 2009. *Deep South: A Social Anthropological Study of Caste and Class*. Columbia: University of South Carolina Press.

De Boeck, Filip. 2012. "Infrastructure: Commentary from Filip De Boeck; Contributions from Urban Africa towards an Anthropology of Infrastructure." Cultural Anthropology website, last modified November 26, 2015. http://www.culanth.org/curated_collections/11-infrastructure/discussions/7-infrastructure-commentary-from-filip-de-boeck.

Deleuze, Gilles. 1995. *Negotiations*. Translated by Martin Joughin. New York: Columbia University Press.

Deloria, Vine. 1969. *Custer Died for Your Sins: An Indian Manifesto*. New York: Macmillan.

Denzin, N. K., and Y. S. Lincoln. 1994. "Introduction: Entering the Field of Qualitative Research." In *Handbook of Qualitative Research*, edited by N. K. Denzin and Y. S. Lincoln, 1–17. Thousand Oaks CA: SAGE.

Dermer, Alicia. 2004. "Loss of Antioxidants in Breastmilk: What Is the Clinical Relevance?" *Archives of Diseases in Childhood: Fetal Neonatal Edition* 89 (6): F518–20.

DeSoucey, Michaela. 2016. *Contested Tastes: Foie Gras and the Politics of Food*. Princeton: Princeton University Press.

Dettwyler, Katherine A. 1998. "More Than Nutrition: Breastfeeding in Urban Mali." *Medical Anthropology Quarterly* 2 (2): 172–83.

Diamond, Jared. 1995. "Father's Milk: From Goats to People, Males Can Be Mammary Mammals, Too." *Discover*, February. http://discovermagazine.com/1995/feb/fathersmilk468.

Diderot, Denis. 1765. "Nourrice." In *Encyclopédie ou Dictionnaire raisonné des sciences, des arts et des métiers*. Paris: André le Breton, Michel-Antoine David, Laurent Durand, Claude Briasson.

Douglas, Mary. 1966. *Purity and Danger: An Analysis of Concepts of Pollution and Taboo*. London: Routledge.

Draper, Susan B. 1996. "Breast-Feeding as a Sustainable Resource System." *American Anthropologist* 98 (2): 258–65.

DuBois, W. E. B. 1939. *Black Folk Then and Now: An Essay in the History and Sociology of the Negro Race*. New York: Holt.

Ebrahim, G. J. 1980. *Breast Feeding: The Biological Option*. New York: Schocken Books.

Edelman, Marc. 2001. "Social Movements: Changing Paradigms and Forms of Politics." *Annual Review of Anthropology* 30:285–317.

Eidelman, Arthur I., and Richard J. Schanler. 2012. "Policy Statement on Breastfeeding and the Use of Human Milk." *Pediatrics* 129 (3): e827–41.

El Guindi, Fadwa. 2011. "Kinship by Suckling: Extending Limits on Alliance in Endogamous Systems." *Anthropological Forum–Peter the Great Museum of Anthropology and Ethnography (Kunstkamera), Russian Academy of Sciences* (Special Forum on Kinship) 15:381–84.

———. 2012. "Blood and Milk." *Anthropos* 107:545–55.

Ellingson, Laura. L., and Carolyn Ellis. 2008. "Autoethnography as Constructionist Project." In *Handbook of Constructionist Research*, edited by J. A. Holstein and J. F. Gubrium, 445–66. New York: Guilford Press.

Ellis, Carolyn. 2004. *The Ethnographic I: A Methodological Novel about Autoethnography*. Walnut Creek CA: AltaMira Press.

Ellis, Carolyn, and Arthur P. Bochner. 2000. "Autoethnography, Personal Narrative, Reflexivity: Researcher as Subject." In *The Handbook of Qualitative Research*, edited by N. Denzin and Y. Lincoln, 733–68. Thousand Oaks CA: SAGE.

Ellison, Marcia A. 2003. "Authoritative Knowledge and Single Women's Unintentional Pregnancies, Abortions, Adoption, and Single Motherhood: Social Stigma and Structural Violence." *Medical Anthropology Quarterly* 17 (3): 322–47.

Elyacher, J. 2010. "Phatic Labor, Infrastructure, and Questions of Empowerment." *American Ethnologist* 37 (3): 452–64.

Enke, Anne. 2007. *Finding the Movement: Sexuality, Contested Space, and Feminist Activism*. Durham: Duke University Press.

Faircloth, Charlotte. 2009. "Mothering as Identity-Work: Long-Term Breastfeeding and Intensive Motherhood." *Anthropology News* 50 (2): 15–17.

———. 2013. *Militant Lactivism? Attachment Parenting and Intensive Motherhood in the UK and France*. London: Berghahn.

Falls, Susan. 2008. "Diamond Signs: Generic Stones & Particular Gems." *Social Semiotics* 18 (4): 449–65.

———. 2014. *Clarity, Cut, and Culture: The Many Meanings of Diamonds*. New York: New York University Press.

———. 2015. "Material Culture Studies." In *Concise Encyclopedia of Consumption and Consumer Studies*, edited by J. Michael Ryan, 414–16. Oxford: Wiley-Blackwell.

Farmer, Paul. 1988. "Bad Blood, Spoiled Milk: Bodily Fluids as Moral Barometers in Rural Haiti." *American Ethnologist* 15 (1): 62–86.

Fildes, Valerie. 1987. *Breast, Bottles, and Babies: A History of Infant Feeding*. Edinburgh: Edinburgh University Press.

Finka, A. E., G. Finka, H. Wilsona, J. Benniea, S. Carrolla, and H. Dicka. 1992. "Lactation, Nutrition and Fertility and the Secretion of Prolactin and Gonadotrophins in Mopan Mayan Women." *Journal of Biosocial Science* 24 (1): 35–52.

Foster, Hal. 1996. "The Artist as Ethnographer." In *The Return of the Real*, 302–9. Cambridge MA: MIT Press.

Fouts, Hillary N., Barry S. Hewlett, and Michael E. Lamb. 2012. "A Biocultural Approach to Breastfeeding Interactions in Central Africa." *American Anthropologist* 114 (1): 123–36.

Fraser, Nancy. 1992. "Rethinking the Public Sphere: A Contribution to the Critique of Actually Existing Democracy, Habermas, and the Public Sphere." In *Habermas and the Public Sphere*, edited by C. Calhoun, 109–42. Cambridge MA: MIT Press.

Friedmann, John. 1992. *Empowerment: The Politics of Alternative Development*. London: Blackwell.

Gell, Alfred. 1998. *Art and Agency: An Anthropological Theory*. Oxford: Clarendon Press.

Geraghty, Sheela R., Kelly A. McNamara, Chelsea E. Dillon, Joseph S. Hogan, Jesse J. Kwiek, and Sarah A. Keim. 2013. "Buying Human Milk via the Internet: Just a Click Away." *Breastfeed Medicine* 8 (6): 474–78. doi:10.1089/bfm.2013.0048.

Giles, Fiona. 2003. *Fresh Milk*. New York: Simon and Schuster.

———. 2010. "From 'Gift of Loss' to Self Care: The Significance of Induced Lactation in Takashi Miike's *Visitor Q*." In *Giving Breastmilk: Body Ethics and Contemporary Breastfeeding Practice*, edited by Rhonda Shaw and Alison Bartlett, 236–49. Toronto: Demeter Press.

Giuliani, Francesca, Ilaria Rovelli, Chiara Peila, Stefana Liguori, Enrico Bertino, and Alessandra Coscia. 2014. "Donor Milk: Current Perspectives." *Research and Reports in Neonatology* 4:125–30.

Golden, Janet. 1996. "From Commodity to Gift: Gender, Class, and the Meaning of Breast Milk in the Twentieth Century." *The Historian* 59:1–9.

Goldin, Claudia. 2006. "The Quiet Revolution That Transformed Women's Employment, Education, and Family." *American Economic Association Papers and Proceedings* 96 (2): 1–21.

Goldschmidt, Walter. 1955. "Social Class and the Dynamics of Status in America." *American Anthropologist* 57 (6): 1209–17.

Goodman, Percival, and Paul Goodman. 1960. *Communitas: Means of Livelihood and Ways of Life*. New York: Vintage.

Gottdeiner, Mark. 1995. *Postmodern Semiotics: Material Culture and the Forms of Postmodern Life*. Oxford: Blackwell.

Gottschang, Suzanne Zhang. 2007. "Maternal Bodies, Breast-Feeding, and Consumer Desire in Urban China." *Medical Anthropology Quarterly* 21 (1): 64–80.

Graham-Harrison, Emma. 2014. "UAE Law Requires Mothers to Breastfeed for First Two Years." *The Guardian*, February 7, 03.55 EST, Middle East. http://www.theguardian.com/world/2014/feb/07/uae-law-mothers-breastfeed-first-two-years.

Gras-Le, G., D. Lepelletier, T. Debillon, V. Gournay, E. Espaze, and J. Roze. 2003. "Contamination of a Milk Bank Pasteuriser Causing a *Pseudomonas aeruginosa* Outbreak in a Neonatal Intensive Care Unit." *Archives of Disease in Childhood, Fetal and Neonatal Edition* 88 (5): F434–35. doi:10.1136/fn.88.5.F434.

Gribble, Karleen D. 2014. "Perception and Management of Risk in Internet-Based Peer-to-Peer Milk-Sharing." *Early Child Development and Care* 84 (1): 84–98. doi:10.1080/03004430.2013.772994.

Griswold, Zara. 2005. *Surrogacy Was the Way: Twenty Intended Mothers Tell Their Stories*. Gurnee IL: Nightengale Press.

Guillemeau, Jacques. 1612. *The Nursing of Children*. London: A. Hatfield.

Habermas, Jürgen. (1962) 1989. *The Structural Transformation of the Public Sphere: An Inquiry into a Category of Bourgeois Society*. Translated by Thomas Burger with Frederick Lawrence. Cambridge MA: MIT Press.

Haiven, Max, and Alex Khasnabish. 2014. *The Radical Imagination*. London: Zed Books.

Halle, David. 1994. *Inside Culture: Art and Class in the American Home*. Chicago: University of Chicago Press.

Hanna, N., K. Ahmed, M. Anwar, A. Petrova, M. Hiatt, and T. Hegyi. 2004. "Effect of Storage on Breast Milk Antioxidant Activity." *Archives of Diseases in Childhood: Fetal Neonatal Edition* 89 (6): F518–20.

Haraway, Donna. 1998. "Living Images: Conversations with Lynn Randolph." In *Millennial Myths: Paintings by Lynn Randolph*. Tempe: Arizona State University Art Museum.

———. 2013. Skype interview by Rick Dolphijn, June 29. Department of Media and Culture Studies, Faculty of Humanities, Utrecht University. https://www.youtube.com/watch?v=CNekH7S3Jhg.

Harvey, Penny, and Hannah Knox. 2015. *Roads: An Anthropology of Infrastructure and Expertise*. Ithaca: Cornell University Press.

Hayano, David. 1979. "Auto-Ethnography: Paradigms, Problems and Prospects." *Human Organization* 38 (1): 99–104.

Haynes, Todd, dir. 1991. *Poison*. Zeitgeist Films.

Hays, K. Michael. 1984. "Critical Architecture: Between Culture and Form." *Perspecta* 21:14–29.

Helmreich, Stefan. 2008. "Species of Biocapital." *Science as Culture* 17 (4): 463–78.

Hemingway, Ernest. 1930. *In Our Time*. New York: Charles Scribner.

Herdt, Gilbert. 2005. *The Sambia: Ritual, Sexuality, and Change in Papua New Guinea*. 2nd ed, New York: Wadsworth.

Hicks, Dan, and M. C. Beaudry, eds. 2010. *The Oxford Handbook of Material Culture Studies*. Oxford: Oxford University Press.

HMBANA. 2014. "Human Milk Banking Association of North America Takes a Stand against Paying for Donations. *HMBANA Matters* (9):2–3.

HM4HB. 2015. "Georgia HM4HB Facebook Administrator Reminder." Last modified May 11.

Hogan, Susan. 2008. "Breast and the Beestings: Rethinking Breastfeeding Practices, Maternity Rituals and Maternal Attachment in Britain and Ireland." *Journal of International Women's Studies* 10 (2): 141–60.

Holmes, Megan. 1997. "Disrobing the Virgin: The *Madonna Lactans* in Fifteenth-Century Florentine Art." In *Picturing Women in Renaissance and Baroque Italy*, edited by Geraldine A. Johnson and Sara F. Mathews Grieco, 167–95. New York: Cambridge University Press.

Hunt, S., and N. Junco. 2006. "Introduction to Two Thematic Issues: Defective Memory and Analytical Autoethnography." *Journal of Contemporary Ethnography* 35 (4): 371–72.

Ingold, Tim. 2008. "When ANT Meets SPIDER: Social Theory for Arthropods." In *Material Agency: Towards a Non-Anthropocentric Approach*, edited by Carl Knappett and Lambros Malafouris, 209–15. London: Springer.

———. 2013. *Making: Anthropology, Archaeology, Art and Architecture*. London: Routledge.

Ip, Stanley, Mei Chung, Gowri Raman, Priscilla Chew, Nombulelo Magula, Deirdre DeVine, Thomas Trikalinos, and Joseph Lau. 2007. *Breastfeeding and Maternal and Infant Health Outcomes in Developed Countries*, edited by the U.S. Department of Health and Human Services. Rockville MD: Agency for Healthcare Research and Quality.

Jelliffe, E. 1976. "Maternal Nutrition and Lactation." In *Breastfeeding and the Mother*, 119–43. Amsterdam: Elsevier.

Jodorowsky, Alejandro, with Gilles Farcet. 2009. *Sacred Trickery and the Way of Kindness: The Radical Wisdom of Jodo*. Translated by Ariel Godwin. Rochester VT: Inner Traditions.

Jones, Stacy. 2005. "(M)othering Loss: Telling Adoption Stories, Telling Performativity." *Text and Performance Quarterly* 25 (2): 113–35.

Jorrisen, Joanne. 2007. "Literature Review: Outcomes Associated with Postnatal Exposure to Polychlorinated Biphenyls (PCBS) via Breast Milk." *Advances in Prenatal Care* 7 (5): 230–37.

Jung, Courtney. 2015. "Overselling Breast-Feeding." *New York Times*, October 16, Opinion. http://www.nytimes.com/2015/10/18/opinion/sunday /overselling-breast-feeding.html?action=click&pgtype=Homepage& module=opinion-c-col-right-region&region=opinion-c-col-right-region& WT.nav=opinion-c-col-right-region&_r=0.

Juris, Jeffrey S. 2012. "Reflections on #Occupy Everywhere: Social Media, Public Space, and Emerging Logics of Aggregation." *American Ethnologist* 39 (2): 259–79.

Kaufman, Sharon, Ann Russ, and Janet Shim. 2006. "Aged Bodies and Kinship Matters." *American Ethnologist* 33 (1): 81–99.

Keaton, Buster, dir. 1925. *Go West*. Buster Keaton/Metro-Goldwyn Productions.

Keim, Sarah, Joseph Hogan, Kelly McNamara, Vishnu Gudimetla, Chelsea Dillon, Jesse Kwiek, and Sheela Geraghty. 2013. "Microbial Contamination of Human Milk Purchased via the Internet." *Pediatrics* 132 (5): e1227–35. doi:10.1542/peds.2013-1687.

Keim, Sarah, K. A. McNamara, C. M. Jayadeva, A. C. Braun, C. E. Dillon, and S. R. Geraghty. 2014. "Breast Milk Sharing via the Internet: The Practice and Health and Safety Considerations." *Maternal and Child Health Journal* 18 (6): 1471–49. doi:10.1007/s10995-013-1387-6.

Keim, Sarah, Manjusha M. Kulkarni, Kelly McNamara, Sheela R. Geraghty, Rachael M. Billock, Rachel Ronau, Joseph S. Hogan, and Jesse J. Kwiek. 2015. "Cow's Milk Contamination of Human Milk Purchased via the Internet." *Pediatrics* 135 (5): e1157–62. doi:10.1542/peds.2014-3554.

Kelley, Heidi, and Ken Betsalel. 2004. "Mind's Fire: Language, Power, and Representations of Stroke." *Anthropology and Humanism* 29 (2): 104–16.

Kennedy, Justice Anthony. 2015. Obergefell v. Hodges. No. 14-556 (U.S. June 26).

Khatib-Chahidi, Jane. 1992. "Milk Kinship in Shi'ite Islamic Iran." In *The Anthropology of Breast-Feeding: Natural Law or Social Construct*, edited by Vanessa Maher, 109–32. New York: Berg.

Klee, Paul. 2014. *Paul Klee: Creative Confession and Other Writings*. Edited by Matthew Gale. London: Tate Museum.

Kolocotroni, Vassaliki, Jane Goldman, and Olga Taxidou, eds. 1999. *Modernism: An Anthology of Sources and Documents*. Chicago: University of Chicago Press.

Koolhaas, Rem, Todd Reisz, Michaal Gergawi, Bimal Mendis, and Tabitha Decker. 2010. "Al Manakh Gulf Continued." *Volume* 23 (April): 1–536.

Kopytoff, Igor. 1986. "The Cultural Biography of Things: Commoditization as Process." In *The Social Life of Things*, edited by Arjun Appadurai, 66–94. Cambridge: Cambridge University Press.

Kristeva, Julia. 1982. *Powers of Horror: An Essay on Abjection*. Translated by Leon S. Roudiez. New York: Columbia University Press.

Kroeker, Lena, and Alyx Beckwith. 2011. "Safe Infant Feeding in Lesotho in the Era of HIV/AIDS." *Annals of Anthropological Practice* 35 (1): 50–66.

Kubrick, Stanley, dir. 1971. *A Clockwork Orange*. Warner Brothers.

La Leche League. 2015. "What Is the Difference between Foremilk and Hindmilk?" La Leche League International, accessed October 15, 2015. http://www.llli.org/faq/foremilk.html.

Langreth, Robert, and Alex Nussbaum. 2011. "Bacteria Tied to Baby's Death Linked to Formula since 1980s." Bloomberg Business News, accessed April 4, 2015. http://www.bloomberg.com/news/articles/2011-12-28/bacteria -tied-to-baby-s-death-has-been-linked-to-formula-since-1980s.

Larkin, Brian. 2008. *Signal and Noise: Media, Infrastructure, and Urban Culture in Nigeria*. Durham: Duke University Press.

———. 2013. "The Politics and Poetics of Infrastructure." *Annual Reviews of Anthropology* 42:327–43.

Law, John. 2009. "The Materials of STS." Version of April 9, accessed December 1, 2015. http://www.heterogeneities.net/publications /Law2008MaterialsofSTS.pdf.

Leinard, Pierre. 2010. "Disgust, Habit or ?: The Evolution of Avoidance." American Anthropological Association Annual Conference, November 17–21, New Orleans.

Lesser, Alexander. 1933. *The Pawnee Ghost Dance Hand Game: A Study in Cultural Change*. New York: Columbia University.

Lewin, Tamar. 2014. "Coming to U.S. for Baby, and Womb to Carry It: Foreign Couples Heading to America for Surrogate Pregnancies." *New York Times*, July 6, A1, Business.

Lingis, Alphonso. 2004. *Trust*. Minneapolis: University of Minnesota Press.

Lockrem, Jessica, and Adonio Lugo. 2011. "Infrastructure." *Cultural Anthropology* 26 (4). http://www.culanth.org/curated_collections/11-infrastructure.

Lopez, Ricardo. 2013. "Prolacta Develops Niche Delivering Breast Milk to Hospitals." *Los Angeles Times*, October 23, Business. http://www.latimes .com/business/la-fi-breast-milk-processing-20131025-story.html-page=1.

Lothario de Segni, Cardinal-Deacon (Pope Innocent III). 1190–98. *On the Misery of the Human Condition* (Treatise). Rome, Italy. Retrieved at http:// www.montville.net/cms/lib3/NJ01001247/Centricity/Domain/825/On %20the%20Misery%20of%20the%20Human%20Condition.pdf.

Lunceford, Brett. 2012. "Weaponizing the Breast: Lactivism and Public Breastfeeding." In *Naked Politics: Nudity, Political Action, and The Rhetoric of the Body*, 35–80. Lanham MD: Lexington Books.

Lynd, Robert S., and Helen M. Lynd. 1929. *Middletown: A Study in Contemporary American Culture*. New York: Harcourt, Brace.

Mabilia, Mara. 2005. *Breast Feeding and Sexuality: Behaviour, Beliefs, and Taboos among the Gogo Mothers in Tanzania*. New York: Berghahn Books.

MacClancy, Jeremy. 2003. "The Milk Tie." *Anthropology of Food*, September. http://aof.revues.org/339.

Maharawal, Manissa. 2013. "From Safer Spaces to Affective Politics: The Case of the Free University." Presentation at the American Anthropological Association Annual Conference, November 20–24, Chicago.

Maher, Vanessa, ed. 1992. *The Anthropology of Breast-Feeding: Natural Law or Social Construct*. New York: Berg.

Malinowski, Bronislaw. (1922) 1984. *Argonauts of the Western Pacific: An Account of Native Enterprise and Adventure in the Archipelagoes of Melanesian New Guinea*. Long Grove IL: Waveland Press.

Manes, Yael. 2011. *Motherhood and Patriarchal Masculinities in Sixteenth-Century Italian Comedy*. Farnham UK: Ashgate.

Marcus, George E., and Michael M. J. Fischer. 1986. *Anthropology as Cultural Critique: An Experimental Moment in the Human Sciences*. Chicago: University of Chicago Press.

Maréchal, Garance. 2010. "Autoethnography." In *Encyclopedia of Case Study Research*, edited by G. Durepos and E. Wiebe A. J. Mills. Thousand Oaks CA: SAGE.

Martin, Andrew. 2008. "Melamine Traces Found in U.S. Infant Formula." *New York Times*, November 25, A19. http://www.nytimes.com/2008/11/26/us/26formula.html?_r=0.

Martin, Courtney, and John Cary. 2014. "Shouldn't the Breast Pump Be as Elegant as an iPhone and as Quiet as a Prius by Now?" (blog entry). *Motherlode*, NYTimes.com, March 16. http://parenting.blogs.nytimes.com/2014/03/16/shouldnt-the-breast-pump-be-as-elegant-as-an-iphone-and-as-quiet-as-a-prius-by-now/?_r=0.

Maskovsky, Jeff. 2013a. "Critical Anthropologies of the United States." In *Handbook of Sociocultural Anthropology*, edited by James Carrier and Deborah Gewertz. New York: Bloomsbury Press.

Maskovsky, Jeff. 2013b. "Protest Anthropology in a Moment of Global Unrest." *American Anthropologist* 115 (1): 126–29.

Maskovsky, Jeff, and Ida Susser, eds. 2009. *Rethinking America: The Imperial Homeland in the 21st Century*. Boulder CO: Paradigm Publishers.

Matorras, R. 2005. "Reproductive Exile versus Reproductive Tourism." *Human Reproduction* 20 (12): 3571. doi:10.1093/humrep/dei223. PMID 16308333.

Mauss, Marcel. (1925) 2016. *The Gift*. Selected, Annotated, and Translated by Jane I. Guyer. Expanded ed. Chicago: HAU Books, distributed by the University of Chicago Press.

McCloud, Scott. 1994. *Understanding Comics: The Invisible Art*. New York: William Morrow.

McCulloch, Warren S. 1945. "A Heterarchy of Values Determined by a Topology of Nervous Nets." *Bulletin of Mathematical Biophysics* 7:89–93.

Mead, M. Nathaniel. 2008. "Contaminants in Human Milk: Weighing the Risks against the Benefits of Breastfeeding." *Environmental Health Perspectives* 116 (10): A426–34.

Meek, Joan. 2001. "Breastfeeding in the Workplace." *Pediatric Clinics of North America* 48:461–74.

Merleau-Ponty, Maurice. 1964. "Eye and Mind." In *The Primacy of Perception*, edited by James E. Edie, 159–90. Evanston IL: Northwestern University Press.

Mesch, Claudia, and Viola Michely, eds. 2007. *Joseph Beuys: The Reader*. Cambridge MA: MIT Press.

Meyers, Fred, ed. 2002. *The Empire of Things: Regimes of Value and Material Culture*. Santa Fe NM: SAR Press.

Miller, Elizabeth M., Marco O. Aiello, Masako Fujita, Katie Hinde, Lauren Milligan, and E. A. Quinn. 2013. "Field and Laboratory Methods in Human Milk Research." *American Journal of Human Biology* 25 (1): 1–11.

Miller, George, dir. 2015. *Mad Max: Fury Road*. Warner Brothers.

Miner, Horace. 1956. "Body Ritual among the Nacirema." *American Anthropologist* 58:503–7.

Mol, Annemarie. 2003. *The Body Multiple: Ontology in Medical Practice*. Durham: Duke University Press.

Morton, Timothy. 2013. *Hyperobjects: Philosophy and Ecology after the End of the World*. Minneapolis: University of Minnesota Press.

Nguyen, Vinh-Kim. 2010. *The Republic of Therapy: Triage and Sovereignty in West Africa's Time of AIDS*. Durham: Duke University Press.

Obladen, Michael. 2012. "Guttus, Tralatte and Téterelle: A History of Breast Pumps." *Journal of Perinatal Medicine* 40 (6): 669–75. doi:10.1515/jpm -2012-0120.

Osborn, M. S. 1979. "The Rent Breasts, Part II." *Midwife, Health Visitor & Community Nurse* 15 (9): 347–48.

Pallasmaa, Juhani. 2012. *The Eyes of the Skin: Architecture and the Senses*. 3rd ed. Padstow UK: Wiley and Sons.

Palmquist, Aunchalee. 2015. "Demedicalizing Breast Milk: The Discourses, Practices, and Identities of Informal Milk Sharing." In *Ethnographies of*

Breastfeeding: Cultural Contexts and Confrontations, edited by T. Cassidy and A. El Tom, 23–44. New York: Bloomsbury Press.

Palmquist, Aunchalee, and Kirsten Doehler. 2014. "Contextualizing Online Human Milk Sharing: Structural Factors and Lactation Disparity among Middle Income Women in the U.S." *Social Science & Medicine* 122:140–47.

———. 2016. "Human Milk Sharing Practices in the U.S." *Maternal & Child Nutrition* 12 (12): 278–90.

Panczuk, Julia, Sharon Unger, Deborah O'Connor, and Shoo Lee. 2014. "Human Donor Milk for the Vulnerable Infant: A Canadian Perspective." *International Breastfeeding Journal* 9 (4). doi:10.1186/1746-4358-9-4.

Papanek, Victor. 1971. *Design for the Real World: Human Ecology and Social Change.* New York: Pantheon Books.

Parkes, Peter. 2004. "Fosterage, Kinship, and Legend: When Milk Was Thicker Than Blood?" *Comparative Studies in Society and History* 46 (3): 587–615.

———. 2005. "Milk Kinship in Islam: Substance, Structure, History." *Social Anthropology* 13 (3): 307–29.

Paxton, Heather. 2010. "Locating Value in Artisan Cheese: Reverse Engineering Terroir for New-World Landscapes." *American Anthropologist* 112 (3): 444–57. doi: 10.1111/j.1548-1433.2010.01251.x.

———. 2012. *The Life of Cheese: Crafting Food and Value in America.* Berkeley: University of California Press.

Peirano, Mariza G. S. 1998. "When Anthropology Is at Home: The Different Contexts of a Single Discipline." *Annual Review of Anthropology* 27:105–28.

Peirce, Charles Sanders. 1931–58. *Collected Writings.* Edited by Charles Hartshorne, Paul Weiss, and Arthur W. Burks. 8 vols. Cambridge MA: Harvard University Press.

Pew Research Center. 2011. "America's Muslim Population 2030." Pew Research Center, accessed April 21, 2015. http://www.pewresearch.org/daily-number/americas-muslim-population-2030.

Pollack, Andrew. 2015. "Breast Milk Becomes a Commodity, with Mothers Caught Up in Debate." *New York Times,* March 20. http://www.nytimes.com/2015/03/21/business/breast-milk-products-commercialization.html?mtrref=undefined&gwh=5259916434BE62551AEDD1F39C5BF0B1&gwt=pay&assetType=nyt_now.

Powdermaker, Hortense. 1939. *After Freedom: A Cultural Study in the Deep South.* New York: Viking Press.

———. 1950. *Hollywood, the Dream Factory: An Anthropologist Looks at the Movie-Makers.* Boston: Little, Brown.

Prown, Jules David. 2001. "Material Culture: Can the Farmer and the

Cowman Still Be Friends?" In *Art as Evidence: Writings on Art and Material Culture*, 235–42. New Haven: Yale University Press.

Radin, Margaret Jane. 2001. *Contested Commodities*. Cambridge MA: Harvard University Press.

Rancière, J. 2010. *Dissensus: On Politics and Aesthetics*. New York: Continuum.

Randolph, Lynn. 2010. "Modest Witness: A Painter's Collaboration with Donna Haraway." LynnRandolph.com, accessed March 2, 2015. http://www.lynnrandolph.com/ModestWitness.html.

Raphael, Dana. 1955. *The Tender Gift: Breastfeeding*. New York: Schocken Books.

Reed-Danahay, Deborah. 1997. *Auto/ethnography: Rewriting the Self and the Social*. London: Bloomsbury Academic.

Relethford, John. 2012. *The Human Species: An Introduction to Biological Anthropology*. 9th ed. New York: McGraw-Hill.

Reyes-Foster, Beatriz, Shannon Carter, and Melanie Sberna Hinojosa. 2015a. "Milk Sharing in Practice: A Descriptive Analysis of Peer Breastmilk Sharing." *Breastfeeding Medicine* 10 (5): 263–69.

Reyes-Foster, Beatriz, Shannon Carter, and Tiffany Rogers. 2015b. "Liquid Gold or Russian Roulette? Risk and Human Milk Sharing in the US News Media." *Health Risk & Society* 17 (1): 30–45.

Rivers, W. H. R. 1913. *Report on Anthropological Research Outside America*. Edited by W. H. R. Rivers, A. E. Jenks, and S. G. Morley. Washington DC: Carnegie Institution.

Robb, Alice. 2014. "Bring Back the Wet Nurse! A Solution for Working Mothers That Has Been Around for Centuries." *New Republic*, last modified July 22. http://www.newrepublic.com/article/118786/breastfeeding-wet-nurses-mommy-wars.

Rohrer, Ingo. 2013. *Cohesion and Dissolution: Friendship in the Globalized Punk and Hardcore Scene of Buenos Aires*. Wiesbaden: Springer.

Rosin, Hanna. 2009. "The Case against Breast-Feeding." *The Atlantic*, April. http://www.theatlantic.com/magazine/archive/2009/04/the-case-against-breast-feeding/307311/.

Ross, Susan M, ed. 2006. *American Families Past and Present: Social Perspectives on Transformations*. New Brunswick NJ: Rutgers University Press.

Rotenberg, Robert. 2014. "Material Agency in the Urban Material Culture Initiative." *Museum Anthropology* 37 (1): 36–45. doi:10.1111/muan.12048.

Rudd, Elizabeth, and Lara Descartes, eds. 2008. *The Changing Landscape of Work and Family in the American Middle Class*. Lanham MD: Lexington Books.

Ryan, Alan S. 1988. "The Role of Bioanthropology in the Infant Formula Industry: Dietary Iron Status of American Infants." *Central Issues in Anthropology* 7 (2): 39–56.

Sauers, Jenna. 2010. "Photos Reimagine Breast Milk as a High-Fashion Weapon" (blog entry). *Jezebel*, accessed June 1, 2015. goo.gl/UXc7S7.

Schneider, Arnd, and Christopher Wright, eds. 2006. *Contemporary Art and Anthropology*. Oxford: Berg.

———, eds. 2010. *Between Art and Anthropology: Contemporary Ethnographic Practice*. Oxford: Berg.

Schneider, David. 1968. *American Kinship: A Cultural Account*. Chicago: University of Chicago Press.

Sears, William, and Martha Sears. 2001. *The Attachment Parenting Book: A Commonsense Guide to Understanding and Nurturing Your Baby*. Boston: Little, Brown.

Sellen, Daniel W. 2012. "Anthropological Approaches to Understanding the Causes of Variation in Breastfeeding and Promotion of 'Baby Friendly' Communities." *Nutritional Anthropology* 25 (1): 19–29.

Sharp, Lesley A. 2006. *Strange Harvest: Organ Transplants, Denatured Bodies, and the Transformed Self*. Berkeley: University of California Press.

Shaw, Rhonda. 2010. "Perspective on Ethics and Human Milk Banking." In *Giving Breastmilk: Body Ethics and Contemporary Breastfeeding Practice*, edited by Rhonda Shaw and Alison Bartlett, 83–97. Toronto: Demeter Press.

Shaw, Rhonda, and Alison Bartlett, eds. 2010. *Giving Breastmilk: Body Ethics and Contemporary Breastfeeding Practice*. Toronto: Demeter Press.

Schendel, Willem van, and Itty Abraham, eds. 2005. *Illicit Flows and Criminal Things: States, Borders, and the Other Side of Globalization*. Bloomington: Indiana University Press.

Shklovsky, Viktor. (1917) 2004. "Art as Technique." In *Literary Theory: An Anthology*, 5–21. Malden MA: Blackwell.

Simpson, Audra. 2014. *Mohawk Interruptus: Political Life across the Borders of Settler States*. Durham: Duke University Press.

Smith, Stevie. 1936. *Novel on Yellow Paper*. London: Cape.

Sparkes, A. C. 2000. "Autoethnography and Narratives of Self: Reflections on Criteria in Action." *Sport Journal* 17:21–24.

Spiro, Melford. 1955. "The Acculturation of American Ethnic Groups." *American Anthropologist* 57 (6): 1240–52.

Star, Susan Leigh. 1999. "The Ethnography of Infrastructure." *American Behavioral Scientist* 43 (4): 377–91.

Stearns, Cindy. 2010. "The Breast Pump." In *Giving Breastmilk: Body Ethics and Contemporary Breastfeeding Practice*, edited by Rhonda Shaw and Alison Bartlett, 11–23. Toronto: Demeter Press.

Steinbeck, John. 1939. *The Grapes of Wrath*. New York: Viking.

Steiner, Leslie Morgan. 2013. *The Baby Chase: How Surrogacy Is Transforming the American Family*. New York: St. Martin's Press.

Stephen, Michele. 1995. *A'aisa's Gifts: A Study of Magic and the Self*. Berkeley: University of California Press.

Stern, Lesley. 2016. "When I Devour Your Soul, We Are Neither Human nor Animal: Cinema as Animist Universe." *Cine-Files*, Spring (10). http://www.thecine-files.com/once-ive-devoured-your-soul/.

Stevens, Emily, Thelma Patrick, and Rita Pickler. 2009. "A History of Infant Feeding." *Journal of Perinatal Education* 18 (2): 32–39.

Stevens, J., and Sarah Keim. 2015. "How Research on Charitable Giving Can Inform Strategies to Promote Human Milk Donations to Milk Banks." *Journal of Human Lactation* 31 (3): 344–47.

Stewart, Kathleen. 2008. *Ordinary Affects*. Durham: Duke University Press.

Stilwell, Victoria. 2013. "Bodies Double as Cash Machines with U.S. Income Lagging." *Bloomberg Online News*, October 15, Sustainability. http://www.bloomberg.com/news/2013-10-15/bodies-double-as-cash-machines-with-u-s-income-lagging-economy.html.

Stoller, Paul. 2005. *Stranger in the Village of the Sick: A Memoir of Cancer, Sorcery, and Healing*. Boston: Beacon Press.

Strohm, Kiven. 2012. "When Anthropology Meets Contemporary Art: Notes for a Politics of Collaboration." *Collaborative Anthropologies* 5:98–124.

Stuebe, Allison. 2009. "The Risks of Not Breastfeeding for Mothers and Infants." *Reviews in Obstetrics and Gynecology* 2 (4): 222–31.

Stuebe, Allison, K. D. Gribble, and Aunchalee Palmquist. 2014. "Differences between Online Milk Sales and Peer-to-Peer Milk Sharing. (E-letter reply to Keim et al., 'Microbial contamination of human milk purchased via the Internet')." *Pediatrics Digest*, accessed May 15, 2015. http://pediatricsdigest.mobi/content/132/5/e1227/reply.

Susser, Ida. 2001. "Cultural Diversity in the United States." In *Cultural Diversity in the United States*, edited by Ida Susser and Tom Patterson, 3–15. Malden MA: Blackwell.

Swanson, Kara W. 2014. *Banking on the Body: The Market in Blood, Milk, and Sperm in Modern America*. Cambridge MA: Harvard University Press.

Tamaro, Janet. 2005. *So That's What They're For! The Definitive Breastfeeding Guide*. New York: Adam's Media.

Tanabe, R. 2016. "Leon Battista Alberti." *New World Encyclopedia*, accessed November 2016. http://www.newworldencyclopedia.org/p/index.php?title=Leon_Battista_Alberti&oldid=999404.

Taussig, Michael. 2011. *I Swear I Saw This: Drawings in Fieldwork Notebooks, Namely My Own*. Chicago: University of Chicago Press.

Telegraph. 2008. "Swiss Restaurant to Serve Meals Cooked with Human
   Breast Milk: A Swiss Gastronomist Has Stirred a Controversy in the
   Tranquil Alpine Republic after Announcing That He Will Serve Meals
   Cooked with Human Breast Milk." September 17, News. http://www
   .telegraph.co.uk/news/newstopics/howaboutthat/2976181/Swiss
   -restaurant-to-serve-meals-cooked-with-human-breast-milk.html.

Teman, Elly. 2010. *Birthing a Mother: The Surrogate Body and the Pregnant
   Self*. Berkeley: University of California Press.

Thorley, V. 2008. "Sharing Breastmilk: Wet Nursing, Cross Feeding, and Milk
   Donations." *Breastfeed Review* 16 (1): 25–29.

Trounson, Rebecca, and David Ng. 2012. "Lebbeus Woods Dies at 72; Radical
   Architect." *Los Angeles Times,* November 30. http://articles.latimes.com
   /2012/nov/03/local/la-me-lebbeus-woods-20121104.

Turner, Edith. 2011. *Communitas: The Anthropology of Collective Joy*. New
   York: Palgrave Macmillan.

Turner, Victor. 1967. "Symbols in Ndembu Ritual." In *The Forest of Symbols:
   Aspects of Ndembu Ritual*. Ithaca: Cornell University Press.

———. 1969. *The Ritual Process*. Chicago: Aldine.

U.S. Department of Labor. 2010. Fair Labor Standards Act—Break Time for
   Nursing Mothers Provision, section 7(r).

U.S. Surgeon General. 2011. *Surgeon General's Call to Action to Support Breastfeeding*. Rockville MD: U.S. Department of Health and Human Services.

Van Esterik, Penny. 1989. *Beyond the Breast-Bottle Controversy*. New Brunswick NJ: Rutgers University Press.

———. 1992. "Women, Work, and Breastfeeding." *Transactions of the Royal
   Society of Tropical Medicine and Hygiene* 87 (6): 712–804.

———. 2006. *Risks, Rights and Regulations: Communicating about Risk and
   Infant Feeding*. Toronto: National Network on Environments and Women's
   Health, York University.

———. 2009. "Vintage Breast Milk: Exploring the Discursive Limits of
   Feminine Fluids." *Canadian Theatre Review* 137:20–23.

———. 2011. "Genealogies of Nurture: Of Pots and Professors." *Journal of
   Burma Studies* 15 (1): 21–42.

Van Hollen, Cecilia. 2011. "Breast or Bottle? HIV-Positive Women's Responses
   to Global Health Policy on Infant Feeding in India." *Medical Anthropology
   Quarterly* 25 (4): 499–518.

Van Ingen, Philip, and Paul Emmons Taylor, eds. 1912. *Infant Mortality and Milk
   Stations: Special Report Dealing with the Problem of Reducing Infant Mortal-
   ity, Work carried on in Ten Largest Cities in the United States together with
   Details of a Demonstration Held by Private and Public Agencies in New York*

City during 1911 to Determine the Value of Milk Station Work as a Practical Means of Reducing Infant Mortality. New York: New York Milk Committee.

Varughese, Ansa. 2013. "Rob Rhinehart, 24, Creates Soylent: Why You Never Have to Eat Food Again." *Medical Daily*, March 15. http://www.medical daily.com/rob-rhinehart-24-creates-soylent-why-you-never-have-eat-food -again-244648.

Villard, Ray. 2012a. "The Milky Way Contains at Least 100 Billion Planets According to Survey." Hubblesite, January 11. https://web.archive.org /web/20140723213047/http://hubblesite.org/newscenter/archive /releases/2012/07/full/.

———. 2012b. "Milky Way." BBC, March 2. http://web.archive.org/web /20120302071454/http://www.bbc.co.uk/science/space/universe/key _places/milky_way.

Wagner, C. L., D. M. Anderson, and W. B. Pittard. 1996. "Special Properties of Human Milk." *Clinical Pediatrics* 35 (6): 283–93. doi:10.1177 /000992289603500601.

Waldby, Catherine, and Robert Mitchell. 2006. *Tissue Economies: Blood, Organs, and Cell Lines in Late Capitalism*. Durham: Duke University Press.

Waldeck, Sarah. 2002. "Encouraging a Market in Human Milk." *Columbia Journal of Gender and Law* 11 (361).

Walker, Rob. 2015. "Scalies in the Spotlight." *Design Observer*, accessed June 30, 2015. http://designobserver.com/feature/scalies-in-the-spotlight /38849.

Warner, Michael. 2002. *Publics and Counterpublics*. New York: Zone Books.

Warner, W. Lloyd, and Paul S. Lunt. 1941. *The Social Life of a Modern Community*. Yankee City series, vol. 1. New Haven: Yale University Press.

Weaver, Matthew, and Sarah Boseley. 2014. "Liquid Food Linked to Poisoning of Babies Was Sent to 22 Hospitals." *The Guardian*, Health. http://www .theguardian.com/society/2014/jun/05/liquid-food-poisoning-babies -sent-22-hospitals.

Weissman, A. M., B. T. Levy, A. J. Hartz, et al. 2004. "Pooled Analysis of Antidepressant Levels in Lactating Mothers, Breast Milk, and Nursing Infants." *American Journal of Psychiatry* 161:1066–78.

West, Diana, and Lisa Marasco. 2008. *The Breastfeeding Mother's Guide to Making More Milk*. New York: McGraw-Hill.

Whitaker, Elizabeth Dixon. 2000. *Measuring Mamma's Milk: Fascism and the Medicalization of Maternity in Italy*. Ann Arbor: University of Michigan Press.

Whyte, William Foote. 1943. *Street Corner Society: The Social Structure of an Italian Slum*. Chicago: University of Chicago Press

Wickes, J. G. 1953. "A History of Infant Feeding. IV. Nineteenth Century Continued." *Archives of Diseases in Childhood: Fetal Neonatal Edition* 28 (141): 416–22.

Wilk, Richard. 1993. "Altruism and Self Interest: Towards an Anthropological Theory of Decision Making." *Research in Economic Anthropology* 14:191–212.

Wilson, Edward O. 2012. *Social Conquest of the Earth*. New York: Norton.

———. 2013. "The Riddle of the Human Species." *New York Times*, February 24, The Stone. http://nyti.ms/1eENf5W.

Wohlsen, Marcus. 2015. "Cow Milk without the Cow Is Coming to Change Food Forever." *Wired*, last modified April 15. http://www.wired.com/2015/04/diy-biotech-vegan-cheese/.

Wolf, Joan B. 2013. *Is Breast Best? Taking on the Breastfeeding Experts and the New High Stakes of Motherhood*. New York: New York University Press.

Woods, Lebbeus. 1982. *Lebbeus Woods: Aeon, the Architecture of Time; A Monograph*. New York: Express Newspaper.

———. 1989. *OneFiveFour*. New York: Princeton Architectural Press.

———. 1991. *Lebbeus Woods: Terra Nova*. Tokyo: A+U Publishing.

———. 1992. *The New City*. New York: Simon & Schuster.

———. 1993. *War and Architecture = Rat I Arhitektura*. Pamphlet Architecture 15. New York: Princeton Architectural Press.

———. 1997. *Radical Reconstruction*. New York: Princeton Architectural Press.

———. 2008. "LOST AND FOUND" (blog entry). Lebbeus Woods, last modified January 21, 10:51 p.m. https://lebbeuswoods.wordpress.com/2008/01/21/test-3/.

———. 2011. "A Space of Light" (blog entry). Lebbeus Woods, last modified February 15, 3:08 a.m. https://lebbeuswoods.wordpress.com/2011/02/15/a-space-of-light-2/.

———. 2012. "GOODBYE, sort of" (blog entry). Lebbeus Woods, last modified August 11, 10:58 pm. http://lebbeuswoods.wordpress.com/2012/08/11/goodbye-sort-of/.

———, ed. 2015. *Slow Manifesto: Lebbeus Woods Blog*. Edited by Clare Jacobson. New York: Princeton Architectural Press.

World Health Organization. 2009. *Strengthening and Sustaining the Baby-Friendly Hospital Initiative: A Course for Decision-Makers*. WHO, accessed June 20, 2015. http://www.who.int/nutrition/publications/infantfeeding/bfhi_traningcourse_s2/en/.

Yardley, William. 2012. "Lebbeus Woods, Architect, Dies at 72." *New York Times*, November 3, A24.

Yin, R. K. 1989. *Case Study Research: Design and Methods*. Vol. 5. London: SAGE.

Young, Sharon, and Daniel Benyshek. 2010. "Revulsion or Appeal? A Blind Test of the Visual and Olfactory Cues of Human Placental Tissue." American Anthropological Association Annual Conference, November 17–21, New Orleans.

Zeitlyn, Sushila, and Rabeya Rowshan. 1997. "Privileged Knowledge and Mothers' 'Perception': The Case of Breast-Feeding and Insufficient Milk in Bangladesh." *Medical Anthropology Quarterly* 11 (1): 56–68.

Zinn, Howard. 1980. *People's History of the United States*. New York: Harper and Row.

Index

In the Anthropology of Contemporary North America series:

To order or obtain more information on these or other University of Nebraska Press titles, visit nebraskapress.unl.edu.

CPSIA information can be obtained
at www.ICGtesting.com
Printed in the USA
LVOW11s0826210717
542093LV00001B/188/P